THE FIVE STAGES OF MANAGED CARE
Strategies for Providers, HMOs, and Suppliers

Management Series

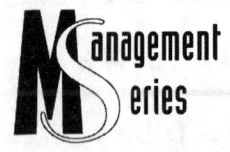

American College of Healthcare Executives
Editorial Board

Austin Ross, FACHE
University of Washington

Jeptha W. Dalston, Ph.D., FACHE
University of Houston

Colene Y. Daniel, CHE
Johns Hopkins Health Systems

William L. Dowling II
Bellingham, Washington

Theodore J. Druhot, FACHE
Hilton Head Island, South Carolina

Diane K. Duin
University of South Dakota

Suzanne M. Garszczynski, Ph.D., CHE
Palmerton Hospital

Paul B. Hofmann, Dr.P.H., FACHE
Alexander and Alexander Consulting Group

Thomas R. Matherlee, FACHE
The Hunter Group

John A. Russell, FACHE
Health Alliance of Pennsylvania

Robert M. Sloane, FACHE
Robert Sloane & Associates

Stuart A. Wesbury, Jr., Ph.D., FACHE
Arizona State University

THE FIVE STAGES OF MANAGED CARE
Strategies for Providers, HMOs, and Suppliers

RUSSELL C. COILE, JR.

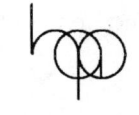

Health Administration Press
Chicago, Illinois

Copyright © 1997 by the Foundation of the American College of Healthcare Executives. Printed in the United States of America. All rights reserved. This book or parts thereof may not be reproduced in any form without written permission of the publisher. Opinions and views expressed in this book are those of the author and do not necessarily reflect those of the Foundation of the American College of Healthcare Executives.

01   00   99   5   4   3

Library of Congress Cataloging-in-Publication Data

Coile, Russell C.
   The five stages of managed care : strategies for providers, HMOs, and suppliers / by Russell C. Coile, Jr.
     p.   cm.—Management Series
   Includes bibliographical references and index.
   ISBN 1-56793-050-6
   1. Health maintenance organizations.   2. Managed care plans (Medical care)   I. Title.
   [DNLM: 1. Managed Care Programs—organization & administration—United States.   2. Practice, Management, Medical—organization & administration—United States. 3. Delivery of Health Care, Integrated—organization & administration—United States.   W 130 AA1 C67f 1996]
RA413.C55   1997
362. 1'0425—dc20
DNLM/DLC
for Library of Congress   96-44119
                                                                           CIP

The paper used in this publication meets the minimum requirements of American National Standard for Information Sciences—Permance of paper for Printed Library materials, ANSI Z39.48—1984. ∞ ™

A Health Administration Press
A division of the Foundation of the
   American College of Healthcare Executives
One North Franklin Street, Suite 1700
Chicago, IL 60606
312/424-2800

*For the past generation, who grew up before HMOs;
my mother and father, Peg Wallace and Russell C. Coile;*

*and to the next generation, my children,
who have always been managed care enrollees,
Courtney and Zachary Coile
and
Amanda and Ariel Angelotti;*

*and to my own healthcare executive, my wife,
Nancy Coile.*

Contents

Preface ix

1 The Five Stages of Managed Care: Organizing for Capitation and Health Reform 1

2 Managed Care Outlook: High Growth and New Markets for HMOs 21

3 Capitation: A New Balance of Power for HMOs and Providers 41

4 Physician-Hospital Strategies for Capitation 61

5 Integrated Delivery Networks: Providers Organize for Managed Care and Direct Contracting 81

6 Primary Care Networks: Integrators of Care in IDNs 101

7 Independent Physician Organizations: Doctor-Owned Medical Networks Put Physicians in Control of Managed Care ... 121

8	Statewide Networks: Providers Organize Mega-Systems to Dominate State Markets . 137
9	Physician-Hospital Integration: Creating New Models of Provider Partnerships 155
10	Provider-Payer Partnerships: Creating the Ultimate Model 177
11	Governing the IDN: New Models for a Post-Reform Environment 195
12	The Sixth Stage of Managed Care: New Models for the Post-Reform Era 209

Index 229

About the Author 253

Preface

THE TRANSFORMATION of U.S. healthcare to a managed care system will be close to complete by the year 2000. Market forces—not government bureaucracy—are driving the conversion from fee-for-service payments to prepaid capitation and managed care. The Clinton health reform plan failed in 1994, but many of the goals of restructuring America's $1 trillion health delivery system are moving forward. The self-reforming healthcare economy results from a convergence of interests among employers, insurers, and healthcare systems (Greenberg 1994).

To hold down health benefit costs, employers have turned to HMOs and managed care insurers who offer low-cost rates. This sets in motion a domino effect that is driving down prices and setting off a rush to integration across the health industry. HMOs and health plans, to keep premiums competitive, have been slashing provider payments and closely controlling service use. Physicians and hospitals are competing for shrinking reimbursement. Suppliers are squeezed by all parties, with little sympathy for the effect of managed care on research or new product development.

INTRODUCING MANAGED CARE

The trend toward cost-management by employers, HMOs, and health plans is loosely defined as "managed care," an aggressive cost-management effort by healthcare purchasers and insurers to limit their health spending. Price discounting, prior authorization, and strict controls on utilization now dominate the provision of hospital and medical services. For providers, the effects are falling

Preface

admissions, slumping patient days, fewer procedures and tests, lower payments, and "downsized" facilities.

The trigger factor in understanding the rise of managed care is the percentage of HMO enrollment. The core strategies for transforming America's health delivery system are drawn from managed care and driven by increasing levels of HMO enrollment, which will transform the nation in the five stages of managed care. The patterns in these sophisticated managed care markets are leading the way toward twenty-first century healthcare.

THE FIVE STAGES OF MANAGED CARE

There are five stages of managed care, with quite predictable market events and strategic responses. At every stage, a new set of relationships evolves among the major players, including physicians and hospitals, HMOs and insurers, and employers and government. That is, at each higher level of managed care penetration, providers, payers, and purchasers restructure their relationships, as the players seek to control their market and their destiny.

The key to the variance in the stages is HMO enrollment. The higher the stage number, the higher the HMO enrollment percentage. Following are the five stages of managed care and their respective HMO penetration percentages.

Stage	HMO Penetration
Stage 1 Can't Spell HMO	Less than 5%
Stage 2 Managed Care Gets Aggressive	5–14%
Stage 3 Managed Care Penetration	15–24%
Stage 4 Managed Competition	25–40%
Stage 5 Post-Reform	Greater than 40%

Further characteristics of each stage will be discussed later in the book.

New patterns often arise in response to HMO moves. This has been demonstrated over and over, in advanced markets on the West Coast and Minneapolis–St. Paul, then washing over the rest of the nation. As of 1994, southern California has 35 percent HMO penetration (Hamer 1994). There are a few places where HMO enrollment is even higher!

Based on HMO enrollment and market penetration, there are more than a dozen Stage 5 markets, according to Minnesota-based InterStudy, which maintains a national database on HMO development. Who is a Stage 5 market? No, it is not Los Angeles, Orange County, or Sacramento. Try Portland, Santa Barbara,

Preface

Tucson, and Rochester, New York. With more than 40 percent HMO membership, these are the most heavily penetrated markets in the nation.

The purpose of *The Five Stages of Managed Care* is to inform the health field about the predictable pattern of HMO growth and managed care development and to outline sustainable strategies for coping with each stage of managed care as it becomes the dominant pattern of American healthcare reimbursement and delivery. Managed care will compel consolidation and integration. Providers, HMOs, and suppliers will share a future. They will need successful integration strategies, or they will be isolated as "vendors" and struggle to survive.

THE TWENTY-FIRST CENTURY HEALTH SYSTEM IS A NETWORK

A managed care future demands new models and strategies. Tomorrow's healthcare system is likely to be a network, not an asset-integrated system. There is not enough capital to purchase every hospital, medical practice, and HMO in America. The debt service would cripple any company, even giants like Columbia/HCA, Blue Cross, or Kaiser. The model of the future is Peter Drucker's "network society" (Drucker 1995). The network is a joint business venture or contractual arrangement to provide health services for a prenegotiated price.

Today, insurers and HMOs have the upper hand, because they "own" the enrollees. That situation is changing, however, as hospitals, physicians, large employers, and government agencies are competing to accept risk and manage enrollees. In twenty-first century healthcare, there will be no one dominant model in a network future. But HMOs may reject provider-sponsored networks and physician-hospital organizations (PHOs), preferring to retain control. This reaction is probably based on certain fears:

- PHOs are too specialist-dominated.
- They are not experienced enough or willing to accept capitation.
- They have no stringent provider credentialing criteria.
- They fail to focus on medical management protocols, such as developing clinical pathways.

The ultimate partnership will link providers and payers in integrated plans that minimize administrative costs and clinical duplication. Creating payer-provider partnerships will not be easy.

Preface

A CONCERN FOR QUALITY

At best, managed care is the process of clinical efficiency that carefully monitors quality. At worst, it is the rationing of care by providers and HMOs whose profits go up as less is done for patients. Ultimately, reducing utilization will hit its limits. HMOs, physicians, and hospitals must realize they can only succeed by sharing a single strategy—optimizing the health of enrollees.

Quality indicators like Health Plan Employer Data and Information Set data are a positive first step in the demonstration of health accountability by providers and health plans. The data must be public, and major purchasers—employers, business coalitions, and governments—must make quality a major criterion in contracting with integrated delivery networks.

TRANSFORMATION THROUGH COOPERATION

The triumph of cooperation over competition would in all likelihood lead to the implementation of needed health reforms. Alignment of purchasers, providers, and third party payers could lead to improved access and moderated expenditures. The appeal for cooperation is based on a multi-stakeholder approach that would establish a durable partnership between all major parties who have an interest in reforming America's $1 trillion health system.

This proposal is not a new "voluntary effort," a revival of the short-lived experiment in health industry price restraint in the mid-1970s following the Nixon administration's round of wage-price controls. A twenty-first century appeal for managed cooperation is based in the belief that, fundamentally, healthcare is as much a social institution as it is a market enterprise. The solution for the excesses of competition, such as surplus capacity and high administrative costs, is to engage in a multiparty cooperative structural reform by all major stakeholders—the public, elected officials, insurers and managed care plans, hospitals, physicians and other health professionals, major and small employers, and governments.

Cooperation extends in all directions in this market-driven vision of national health reform, involving purchasers, providers, consumers, suppliers, and governments. The results of cooperation can be improved levels of health for the population and a strengthening of U.S. competitiveness abroad through a reduction in the drag of health costs.

SOURCES

Drucker, P. 1995. *Managing in a Time of Great Change.* New York: Truman Talley Books/Dutton.

Greenberg, D. S. "Health Reform Is Happening Anyway," *Baltimore Sun*, 23 October 1994, p. B1.

Hamer, R. 1994. "Regional Market Analysis." *InterStudy Competitive Edge*, St. Paul, MN. 4 (1): 1–109.

CHAPTER 1

The Five Stages of Managed Care: Organizing for Capitation and Health Reform

Health care reform is dead and buried on Capitol Hill. But the cost-shaving part of it is alive and rampaging across the American landscape as insurers and employers dig in against rising bills.

Daniel S. Greenberg (1994)

WITH THE collapse of the health reform debate, U.S. healthcare providers, HMOs, and suppliers face an uncertain future. Market forces are rapidly filling the vacuum left by Washington's inability to act. Some changes are already evident: declining inpatient use, the substitution of ambulatory care for inpatient care, primary care gatekeeping, consolidation, and integration. Market realities are beginning to hit the healthcare profession, a trend that economists generally applaud. In the mid-1990s, medical care inflation slowed to the lowest annual increase in almost a decade, barely above the rise in consumer prices (Anders 1995; Cochrane 1996). The "economic medicine" HMOs are providing seems to be working.

Economics will drive the future of the health field. As price competition among HMOs intensifies under the managed competition scenario of economic market reforms, the pressure to decrease use of costly hospital care, physician services, and

Five Stages of Managed Care

diagnostic tests will grow stronger. The trigger factor is the decline of HMO premiums, which in 1995 fell 1.2 percent under 1994 price levels—due to pressure from major employers and business coalitions—and which in 1996 fell again by 3.8 percent (Sardinha and Rudd 1994; Cochrane 1996).

The refusal of major employers and government purchasers to pay more is causing a domino effect in healthcare. Buyers are exploiting massive surpluses of virtually every type of provider, facility, and service. The result is a relentless lowering of prices, tougher purchasing policies, and diminishing revenues for the U.S. health industry. The response will be a much-needed restructuring that will affect every hospital, physician, health plan, and supplier in the nation.

The domino effect is particularly evident in markets with high HMO enrollments:

- Major employers aggressively bargain for premium rollbacks from HMOs and insurers.
- The result is that HMOs cannot raise prices and must sometimes accept price cuts.
- Faced with a choice of taking fewer profits, slashing their own administrative costs, or reducing provider payments, the HMOs and insurers recoup most of their losses from providers.
- HMOs employ capitation and micromanage utilization to reduce expenditures for patient care.
- Provider volume (e.g., hospital days and physician referrals) declines sharply.
- Hospitals and physicians have fewer payers to whom they can cost-shift payment cuts to offset the revenue losses from managed care.
- Providers' financial situation is worsened by the government's below-inflation payments from Medicare and below-cost fees from Medicaid.
- Financial pressures force hospital layoffs and widespread restructuring to reduce labor costs by lowering the ratio of professionals to nonprofessionals among the staff.
- Suppliers are relegated to vendor status, competing on price; group purchasing organizations and HMOs demand deeper price cuts; and there is massive consolidation within the healthcare supply chain.

HEALTH REFORM IS AN HMO

Health reform is alive and well in the United States. Market trends—not policy reform—are reshaping the marketplace. If

Hillary Clinton had put the nation's 40 million uninsured out to bid, health reform could have cost only $40 billion to $50 billion dollars, at rates averaging $80 to $100 per member per month, or $1,000 per year.

These are real prices, from Los Angeles, one of the most competitive markets in America. In 1995, CareAmerica, a local HMO, advertised in the *Los Angeles Times* that it was accepting self-employed individuals and families in its HMO, with prices starting at $125 per member per month. In the Sunday issue of the *Times*, Foundation Health Plan advertised its HMO plan with age-specific prices. That monthly premium was competitive with prices elsewhere across the country. In 1994, the average monthly HMO premium was $136 (Hamer 1994a). When California HMOs market to "groups of one" at these prices, the rest of the insurance industry is sure to follow.

Managed care, not federal policy reform, is restructuring the national health system. Congressional policymakers are not going to enact sweeping national reforms, installing "accountable" health plans across the United States. Republican proposals to cut $200 billion to $300 billion in federal health spending by the year 2002 rely heavily on managed care approaches (Georges 1995). Medicaid may be converted into a block grant for states, making it easier for governors to contract with HMOs to handle all care to Medicaid eligibles. Medicare HMOs would be encouraged to assist Congress in reducing Medicare spending from 10 percent annual growth down to 7 percent in five years.

Shifting government health programs to managed care is still controversial. House Speaker Newt Gingrich voiced congressional concerns about managed care in a meeting with the American Medical Association. A senior Republican staffer commented, "Newt is a little schizophrenic on this. The Republicans are as well. They are real skittish about the lack of choice in managed care. But they also know they can't solve the Medicare and Medicaid cost issue without getting more beneficiaries into managed care (quoted in Chen 1995).

THE FIVE STAGES OF MANAGED CARE

American providers and health plans are calculating new strategies and coming swiftly up the learning curve by following the examples of advanced managed care markets. Southern California; Portland, Oregon; Boston, Massachusetts; and Minneapolis–St. Paul are prototypes of competitive managed care markets. There are lessons

Five Stages of Managed Care

to learn and patterns to predict in each of the five stages, especially in the top markets (see Table 1.1). What works, and what fails, can be seen at every one of the five stages of managed care.

Stage 1 markets have little managed care and few pressures to change. Preferred provider organizations are the most common form of managed care plan in these market regions. Most hospitals will organize open-panel physician organizations (independent practice associations), which create a distribution network for discounted patients from health insurers.

In Stage 1 markets, providers should beware of "PHO-itis" in the rush to integration, cautions medical strategist Jonathan T. Lord, M.D., Senior Advisor, Clinical Affairs, of the American Hospital Association in Washington, D.C. Frequent mistakes are (1) the "Y'all come" model of physician organization, with no selection criteria; (2) "$200 in a hat" financing from physicians, which provides little capital or commitment; and (3) the "let's really get an advanced foundation model," an expensive option in states like California that have strong corporate-practice-of-medicine laws (Lord 1994).

Stage 1 has long ago faded in the rearview mirror in many urban markets, especially on the West Coast. Today's Stage 1 markets tend to be more remote and rural. But managed care is finally arriving in

Stage 1. Can't Spell HMO

Characteristics	Strategies
HMO penetration < 5%	Independent HMOs start up
Provider payments	Discounts, prior authorization
Capitation	Bundled prices for specialty care
Indemnity > 30%	Insurers ignore HMOs, develop PPOs
Employers	Install first HMO options
Solo/small groups	Form open-panel independent practice associations
Freestanding hospitals	Prefer to "go it alone"
Ambulatory < 15%	Don't compete with physicians
Profits 6–10%	Invest in capital spending
Quality	Respond to JCAHO, regulation

Examples: Boise, Idaho; El Paso, Texas; Fargo, North Dakota; Ft. Meyers, Florida; Knoxville, Tennessee; Muncie, Indiana; Wilmington, North Carolina

Organizing for Capitation and Health Reform

Table 1.1 Stages of Managed Care: The Top 30 Markets

City	Penetration Rate	Number of HMOs	Dominant Plan
Large Markets			
Portland, Oregon	64%	7	Kaiser
Rochester, New York	63	2	Blue Cross/Blue Shield
San Francisco–Oakland, California	39	17	Kaiser
Minneapolis–St. Paul, Minnesota	39	7	United Health Care
Boston, Massachusetts	36	12	(No dominant)
Los Angeles, California	35	21	Kaiser
San Diego, California	35	11	Kaiser
Sacramento, California	35	10	Kaiser
Salt Lake City, Utah	34	8	(No dominant)
Milwaukee, Wisconsin	31	7	Independent
Medium Markets			
Madison, Wisconsin	61	5	Independent
Stockton, California	53	7	Kaiser
Buffalo, New York	51	3	Independent
Salem, Oregon	50	6	Blue Cross/Blue Shield
Albuquerque, New Mexico	49	5	CIGNA
Albany, New York	48	5	Independent
Santa Barbara, California	46	6	Foundation
Tucson, Arizona	42	5	Independent
Lansing, Michigan	37	3	United Health Care
Providence, Rhode Island	34	5	Harvard Community Health Plan
Small Markets			
Yuba City, California	58	2	Kaiser
Champaign, Illinois	52	3	Two Independents
Dubuque, Iowa	47	2	Independent
Wausau, Wisconsin	37	3	Two Independents
Tallahassee, Florida	36	3	Blue Cross/Blue Shield
Muskegon, Michigan	34	3	United Health Care
Wheeling, West Virginia	34	2	Independent
Waterloo, Iowa	33	1	John Deere Health Plan
Pueblo, Colorado	32	4	Qual Med
Jamestown, New York	30	2	Independent

Source: Adapted from Hamer, R. 1994b. "Regional Market Analysis, Part III." InterStudy Competitive Edge. InterStudy Publications, Bloomington, MN.

states like Alaska, Wyoming, and Montana (Hamer 1996). Managed care penetration is low in Stage 1 markets, but HMO enrollment will rise quickly. Even in Stage 1 markets, aggressive physician management corporations (PMCs) like MedPartners, Caremark, and Phycor, as well as insurance plans and HMOs, are purchasing primary care physician practices throughout the North Central, Southeastern, and Southwest regions (Meyer 1995). Local hospitals are being wooed by Columbia/HCA and nonprofit integrated systems. Few hospitals will be independent by Stage 3.

Strategies for Stage I

It is essential that physicians and hospitals in Stage 1 markets:

- Educate physician leaders and trustees about managed care.
- Develop an open-panel PHO as a fifty-fifty joint venture with physicians and announce plans to close the panel within two years.
- Inform the hospital board that utilization declines and revenue shortfalls will come as managed care grows, and present California data from Stage 3 and Stage 4 markets.
- Undertake hospitalwide cost-containment programs to boost reserves.
- Seek preferred provider designation from insurers and newly arrived HMOs.

Stage 2 markets are often jolted into a later stage by an aggressive act that breaks up historic patterns, like Atlanta's proposed Emory–Columbia/HCA deal. Atlanta, a Stage 2 market in the heart of the South, was stunned by the announcement of a joint venture between Emory University and Columbia/HCA (Rudd 1994a). Although the deal ultimately collapsed, it would have combined Emory's tertiary services and reputation with Columbia/HCA's network of 8 suburban hospitals. The strategy called for Emory's 8 primary care clinics to be consolidated with 19 clinics owned by Columbia/HCA. The bold move by Columbia has accelerated the pace of consolidation between local hospitals and physicians.

A joint venture of this magnitude, involving one of the best-known medical centers in the South, was a jar to the market's equilibrium. But the proposal had a solid business rationale and strategic fit. The combination would have strengthened the position of Columbia/HCA's less prestigious community facilities, and would have provided a feeder network for Emory in Atlanta, a region dominated by larger nonprofit hospitals. A similar transaction later came about in Charleston, South Carolina, between Columbia/HCA and the University of South Carolina Medical Center. The proposal

Stage 2. Managed Care Gets Aggressive

Characteristics	Strategies
HMO penetration 5–15%	HMO contracts with primary care physician (PCP) groups
Provider payments	Deeper discounts, tougher controls
Capitation	First capitation contracts to PCPs
Indemnity < 25%	Hospitals analyze insurer deals
Employers	Form coalitions, share data
Medical groups	Small groups merge, "without walls"
Hospital systems	Purchase weak hospitals
Ambulatory care < 20%	Build medical office buildings to put MDs on campus
Profits 2–3%	Cost containment (but no layoffs)
Quality	Benchmarking

Examples: Charlotte, North Carolina; Indianapolis, Indiana; New Orleans, Louisiana; Omaha, Nebraska; San Antonio, Texas; Topeka, Kansas; York, Pennsylvania

raised a storm of protests from local providers, who were not eager to compete with the new combination of for-profit hospitals and an academic medical center (Cathcart 1995).

Stage 2 markets are especially vulnerable to a Stage 4 move, like Aetna and Prudential acquiring primary care physicians and building staff-model clinics across the South, launching community hospitals into a bidding war to purchase local practices and to recruit physicians for salaried employment. In Stage 2 markets, big-city HMOs arrive in droves, searching for new markets in more thinly populated areas with fewer large employers. In California, midsized cities like Bakersfield, with a population of 566,000, are the focus of intense competition. Kaiser's entry into the Stage 2 Bakersfield market has been challenged by PacifiCare, and others have followed. Small markets like Pueblo, Colorado, has four HMOs competing for a population of only 125,000.

Managed care's erosion of provider payments begins to affect the bottom line in Stage 2. Providers encounter lower prices and more hassles from HMOs. Worse yet, traditional insurers begin to act just as aggressively as HMOs in denying treatment. Busy physicians ignore the slow spread of managed care, discarding those contracts, but younger physicians sign up eagerly. Hospitals are often reluctant to purchase physician practices, not wanting to offend their own key referral sources. Large out-of-area medical groups then take advantage of this hesitancy and begin to acquire primary care physicians (PCPs) themselves.

Once the ground is shifting, hospitals and physicians begin to recognize that managed care's arrival is inevitable, and they begin to prepare. In Houston, a Stage 2 market heading toward Stage 3, a dozen local employers formed the Houston Healthcare Purchasing Organization (HHPO), a collective purchasing coalition that is recruiting as many hospitals as possible into its PPO. Unlike other employer purchasing groups, the Houston employers are placing an early emphasis on quality, not discounts or tough utilization controls. Organizers of the HHPO are focusing on long-term changes in healthcare practices, rather than short-term discounts. Some 45 hospitals are participating in the program, agreeing to be paid on a DRG basis and to submit report-card data. Employers want data to get a true picture of provider performance.

Expect the unexpected in Stage 2, as all parties begin to jockey for position. Providers find the need to cross religious and ownership boundaries to create networks. In Indianapolis, St. Vincent Hospital and Health Care System announced formation of an alliance with Community Hospitals of Indianapolis. The multi-religious partnership would have created a five-hospital network with $900 million in assets. While this alliance was never completed, look for similar such ventures occuring in this stage.

Strategies for Stage 2

The most important strategies that physicians and hospitals can pursue in Stage 2 are:

- Hire a strong medical director who can develop a self-disciplined medical organization.
- Encourage the development of primary care–based medical groups.
- Develop a regional network of preferred hospitals.
- Hire a vice president for managed care to plan and direct strategy.
- Upgrade information systems and purchase software for HMO contract management.
- Educate physician and trustee leadership with site visits to Los Angeles, Albuquerque, or Minneapolis–St. Paul.
- Defer all capital investments for facilities, and save capital for HMO investment and physician organization.

Stage 3. Managed Care Penetration	
Characteristics	**Strategies**
HMO penetration 15–25%	Closed PHO/physician groups
Indemnity < 15%	Drop unprofitable plans
Employers	Direct contracting
Single-specialty groups	Increase primary care groups
Multihospital systems	Merge and expand systems
Ambulatory care < 35%	Satellite ambulatory centers
Profits 2–4%	Staff and management restructuring
Quality	Patient-focused care
Examples: Chicago, Illinois; Boston, Massachusetts; Baltimore, Maryland; Kansas City, Missouri; Hawaii	

Stage 3 markets are chaotic. Old patterns are breaking down, and networking is active, with frequent announcements of new alliances among hospitals, physician groups, and HMOs. In Stage 3, at least one hospital or system will aggressively expand its purchasing of physician groups. Health systems may spend $10 million to $25 million or more to acquire established multispecialty group practices. Insurance companies and HMOs are likely to open their deep pockets in the competition to purchase physicians and develop their company-owned primary care networks.

In Stage 3, network alliances may be easier to negotiate than full mergers when facilities seek partners. In 1994, five Maryland hospitals announced a managed care alliance. St. Agnes Hospital in Baltimore teamed with four suburban facilities, including Northwest Medical Center in Randallstown; the Greater Baltimore Medical Center in Towson; Holy Cross Hospital, located in Silver Spring, a Washington, D.C. suburb; and Montgomery General in Olney. Are five hospitals enough to cover this market of three million? "We don't need a lot of hospitals," explains St. Agnes CEO Robert Pezzoli. "One of the biggest mistakes networks make is that they line up too many hospitals" (Rudd 1994b). More networks are emerging. Johns Hopkins Hospital is forming a seven-hospital network on the hub-and-spoke model, trading on Hopkins' reputation as one of America's leading medical centers.

More crossing of ownership and religious boundaries can be expected in Stage 3 markets. In Phoenix, Arizona, St. Joseph's Hospital and Medical Center is the teaching hub of an eight-hospital alliance with a total of 1,100 beds. The alliance's bylaws were written to ensure that other hospitals would support St. Joseph's mission and would not be involved in sterilization or abortion. In St. Louis, Missouri, Episcopal-sponsored St. Luke's Hospital formed an alliance with three Catholic hospitals. The St. Louis region is emerging as a three-system market, in which the powerful combination of Barnes-Jewish-Christian (BJC Health System) competes with two Catholic-sponsored networks that cannot align because each controls 20 percent of the market (Japsen 1994). Sometimes religious and philosophical differences can be insurmountable. In Portland, Maine, six months of negotiations collapsed when Mercy Hospital, a 200-bed Catholic facility, failed to reach agreement with 598-bed Maine Medical Center and 122-bed Brighton Medical Center. The discussions foundered on the issue of abortions.

Aggressive employers provide managed care momentum in Stage 3 markets. Employers use data on provider performance for direct contracting. In Cleveland, Ohio, a coalition of local employers is demanding hospital data and accelerating the timetable for managed care conversion. Cleveland-area businesses have pushed local hospitals to collect comparable data on costs and quality and to make their performance public. Twenty-nine hospitals organized the Cleveland Health Quality Choice project to collect and present hospital-specific data. The hospitals have released the information on costs and quality, and Cleveland employers—and HMOs—are using the data to handpick hospitals for their networks.

Provider-payer alliances become a game of musical chairs in Stage 3, as health plans use provider performance data to identify preferred partners. In Cleveland, Aetna established itself as one of three major managed care plans in the region, signing up a limited-choice network of 11 Cleveland-area facilities. Aetna priced this "narrow-gate" network fully 25 percent below its 33-hospital plan. Emerald HMO in turn dropped four-hospital Meridia Health System and substituted the Mt. Sinai Medical Center, which scored "particularly well" according to the quality reports (Darby 1994).

Physicians who would not sign up with HMOs in Stages 1 and 2 are, by Stage 3, swamped by HMO controls and sinking revenues. Depression is widespread, and some physicians leave the market. Physician specialists feel the adverse economic effect of managed care. Doctors recognize they must organize to compete. To have leverage in the managed care marketplace requires at least 40 to 75 doctors. Capitation becomes widespread for primary care–based medical groups. The groups develop satellite clinics to serve a wider regional market with thousands of capitated "covered lives."

Specialists merge practices and form local networks, but capitation contracts do not usually come until Stage 4.

Hospitals bring in attorneys to construct physician-hospital organizations in Stage 3. The goals are to integrate managed care contracting and to package physicians for HMO sign-up. PHOs are built in the hope of increasing provider leverage with HMOs to get capitation contracts. Not all physicians want to put their eggs in the hospital basket. The result is physician-sponsored independent practice organizations, (IPOs), which are not owned by any hospital or health system and can negotiate their own deals with HMOs and insurers. Many IPOs will be strategically developed, inviting primary care physicians first. Specialists will be added slowly and selectively.

Strategies for Stage 3

Hospitals must increase the pace of change as they enter Stage 3. Those that fail to create networking and physician strategies now may be left out. Stage 3 hospitals must:

- Develop a regional network of hospitals as a managed care joint venture.
- Capitalize network venture with $10 million to $15 million, and plan to add $5 million to $10 million annually for the next five years.
- Develop a new HMO, or purchase a fifty-fifty joint interest in an existing HMO.
- Close the physician panel and provide performance data on costs and clinical outcomes to all doctors.
- Convert PPOs to HMO point-of-service (POS) models.
- Begin to capitate primary care physician groups or networks.
- Initiate development of clinical paths and standardized medical protocols.
- Tell the board and medical staff to expect that patient days and revenues will fall 15 percent to 25 percent in the next three years.
- Reduce staffing levels and costs quickly as utilization declines.
- Not wait to see if utilization will improve. It won't!

Stage 4 is characterized by "managed competition" over who will control each market's integrated healthcare networks. John Henderson, president of SMG Marketing in Chicago, predicts that by the year 2000, two-thirds of all Americans will be covered by integrated healthcare networks (Henderson 1994).

Five Stages of Managed Care

Stage 4. Managed Competition	
Characteristics	**Strategies**
HMO penetration 25–40%	Regional networks
Indemnity < 5%	Point-of-service (POS) plans
Employers	Purchasing coalitions
Multispecialty groups	Acquire groups or partners
Ambulatory care > 40%	Reduce inpatient beds
Regional hospital networks	Consolidate services
Profits 1–2%	Reengineer clinical care
Quality	Clinical paths/outcomes
Examples: Boston, Massachusetts; Lansing, Michigan; Los Angeles, California; Milwaukee, Wisconsin; Salt Lake City, Utah; San Diego, California; San Francisco–Oakland, California; Tallahassee, Florida	

The competition for control of the networks will put providers into head-to-head competion with HMOs and insurers. The health plans have many advantages in the fight to control networks: They own the enrollees, have deep capital pockets, and bring brand name reputations for marketing. But providers have their own competitive strengths: consumer loyalty, physician-hospital cooperation, and quality service. Aggressive employers provide managed care momentum in Stage 4 markets. San Francisco Bay Area employers have demanded HMO price cuts since 1994 and have won price concessions of 8 to 12 percent. The ripple effect forced HMOs to demand provider payment reductions, setting up the confrontation between managed care plans and providers.

Most Stage 4 markets are located on the West Coast. One of the most ambitious networking efforts took place in California, with the emergence of two nonprofit networks to challenge Kaiser. The first, California Health Network, links San Francisco's California Healthcare System, Sacramento's Sutter Health System, and the Adventist Health System/West, UniHealth, and Loma Linda University Medical Center in the greater Los Angeles area. The second, a Catholic healthcare network, links hospitals affiliated with the Daughters of Charity Health System/West, Catholic Healthcare West, and Scripps in San Diego. Both networks are lining up additional hospitals and physician groups, and may be positioning to develop their own capitated health plan, suggests managed care consultant Peter Boland of Berkeley-based Boland Healthcare (Sardinha and Rudd 1994).

Strategies for Stage 4

At Stage 4, sophisticated hospitals and systems can gain major market advantage from the managed care strategies. To do so, they must:

- Develop joint planning process among network hospitals to begin the process of clinical consolidation on a regional basis.
- Begin to drop from physician panels doctors whose clinical and cost performance is below standard.
- Capitate the hospitals and the specialists.
- Selectively reduce HMO contracts to concentrate on a few key health plans that will contract on partnership terms.
- Expand the scope of patient-centered care reengineering projects and clinical protocols.
- Tighten up cost profiles for the most frequently seen diagnoses and procedures.

Even in Stage 5 markets, the structure of the ultimate integrated delivery system (IDS) is not clear. Competing models are just emerging for the post-reform market. But one thing is evident. In this fifth and final phase of transition, providers will be merging with payers in truly integrated arrangements. SMG Marketing's John Henderson predicts:

- Integration and affiliation will concentrate "seller's power" in dealing with purchasers.
- Emphasis on clinical efficiency and demand reduction will limit costly inpatient services and shift treatment emphasis to ambulatory care and prevention.
- Coordination of care will manage patients for efficiency across a comprehensive continuum of care.
- Integrated delivery systems will use their purchasing clout to form partnerships with suppliers on very cost-effective terms. (Henderson 1994)

Minnesota's Twin Cities of St. Paul and Minneapolis are arguably the most advanced market in America. On the cover of the June 5, 1994, issue of *Hospitals and Health Networks* was a large Minnesota auto license plate: *4 RE4M*. "For reform." The legend on the bottom of the license plate read, "Land of 10,000 HMOs." The Twin Cities are in a post-reform state. Minnesota's legislature adopted a state-level health reform package requiring that every hospital and physician in the state join an integrated service

Five Stages of Managed Care

Stage 5. Post-Reform

Characteristics	Strategies
HMO penetration > 40%	Foundation/equity models
Indemnity 0%	Strengthen POS networks
Employers/coalitions	Purchase on quality
Ambulatory care > 50%	Develop continuum of care
Integrated health networks	Merge with HMO/insurers
Physician mega-groups	Equity/staff models
Profits 2–6%	Manage clinical costs
Quality	Outcomes/patient ratings

Examples: Albuquerque, New Mexico; Buffalo, New York; Madison, Wisconsin; Minneapolis–St. Paul, Minnesota; Portland, Oregon; Rochester, New York; Santa Barbara, California; Tucson, Arizona

---

network (ISN), which would provide services to managed care enrollees, those on Medicare and Medicaid, and the uninsured. Although state legislators are backing off their ambitious plan, one thing is clear about Minnesota: This is HMO territory. Over 40 percent of the Twin Cities population is enrolled in a health maintenance organization (Cerne 1994).

Minnesota providers credit the market—not health reform—for integrating financing and delivery. "The major driver of reform has been the purchasers and their absolute willingness to reward healthcare efficiency and quality," declares George Halvorsen, president of HealthPartners, the Twin Cities' largest HMO. In this advanced market, the three dominant integrated networks are (1) HealthPartners, a staff-model HMO that merged with MedCenters Health Plan, a group-model HMO in 1992; (2) Allina, resulting from a 1994 merger of HealthSpan with the second largest HMO, Medica; and (3) Fairview-HealthEast-University, in partnership with Blue Cross and the Aspen Medical Group of 120 physicians. Consolidation continues to shrink the hospital base, with some predicting a reduction of about 50 percent of current hospital capacity out of the market" (Cerne 1994).

In Stage 5, HMO consolidation has reduced the number of managed care plans, and more mergers are likely in the near future. The 25 largest HMOs in America are prime candidates for mergers, acquisitions, and unfriendly takeovers. Aggressive HMOs like Health Systems International, California's Wellpoint, and a number of Blue Cross plans are sitting on huge capital reserves of hundreds of millions of dollars, which could be used for expansion. Midsized HMOs like Foundation Health, FHP, and PacifiCare may purchase additional small plans, or be acquired by larger ones.

The last element of integrated delivery systems is still to come—the integration of financing and delivery. Many HMOs do not seem ready for full integration, continuing to exploit the surplus of hospitals and doctors. In California, Kaiser Permanente is rethinking its traditional reliance on company-owned hospitals and its own physician group. To save money, Kaiser "could have one-third of our inpatient days out in community hospitals," predicts Ed Carlson, a Kaiser regional vice president (Heimoff 1996, 23). In Stage 5 markets like the Twin Cities, sophisticated employer coalitions are driving the final steps in the integration process. Employers are demanding that HMOs and providers reduce their mutual administrative costs for functions like utilization management, quality assurance, provider credentialing, and network management. When most of the excess utilization has been wrung out of the system by capitation and rigorous cost controls, the last target for cost reduction will be administrative integration.

Strategies for Stage 5

Transition to Stage 5 will be accelerated when state legislatures adopt health reform legislation, such as Medicaid contracting. Systems in Stage 5 should:

- Merge the network with an HMO or insurance company.
- Regionalize all high-technology high-overhead clinical services.
- Close unneeded hospitals, or convert them from acute to continuum of care functions.
- Consolidate physician organizations into one or more multi-specialty group practices.
- Merge the physician organization with the hospital network.
- Eliminate the titles and positions of hospital presidents and replace them with physician or nurse chief operating officers.
- Place all hospitals under a regional executive.
- Complete development of a regional network of ambulatory care centers under the network's "brand name."
- Reconfigure medical office buildings for group practice.
- Conclude the development of clinical paths and treatment protocols for all diagnoses and procedures.

- Complete the computerization of information systems to make them "paperless."
- Identify 10 percent to 15 percent high-risk enrollees for continuous case management.
- Install in-home monitors for chronically ill enrollees.
- Publicly report cost and quality data to enrollees, network providers, purchasers, and the public.
- Develop a new strategic plan for Stage 6.

LOOKING FORWARD: TRANSITIONAL STRATEGIES

What America's hospitals and physicians need are *transitional strategies* to move them through the five stages of managed care. Gerald McManis (1994) observes, "We have some idea of where we would like to be in the year 2000. The question is: What do we do today?" The answer will be different in younger, Stage 2 and Stage 3 markets. As managed care grows nationally, less penetrated markets like Atlanta or Dallas will not take 10 to 15 years to evolve. Stages may last only three to four years in regions with high HMO growth.

Will the integration vehicles of today effectively make the transition to tomorrow? Five years from now, physician-hospital organizations, independent practice associations, foundations, and management service organizations may be relics. New models will emerge, as old structures are merged and modified. A consensus is emerging on the characteristics of successful integrated delivery systems that can survive to Stage 5:

- Capitation will be the dominant form of payment.
- IDSs will serve an enrolled population base of at least 250,000.
- Hospital networks will organize on a regional or statewide basis.
- IDSs will have multi-year, exclusive relationships with insurers and HMOs, and may own a captive HMO or insurer.
- Physician organizations will accept and manage risk under capitation.
- IDSs will provide doctors with shared governance and equity opportunity.
- Systems must manage clinical care to control costs.
- Care managers must have clinical and cost data in "real time" at the point of care. (McManis 1994)

But for every rule of organizing for the next stage of managed development, there will be exceptions. In rural areas, an IDS may serve 25,000 enrollees, not a quarter of a million. Nonprofit and for-profit hospitals may become partners in the same integrated delivery systems. Some HMOs and insurers will own their networks through physician practice acquisition.

On a long-term basis, purchasers will determine the cost and configuration of twenty-first century healthcare in the United States. How much service and technology do consumers want, and how much are they willing to pay? Health Plan A may price its plan low by limiting high-tech care, but provide consumers with ready access to ambulatory services and alternative therapies such as herbal remedies and aromatherapy. Competing HMO B, at the high end of the price spectrum, may offer gamma knives and PET scanners, Ritz-level hospital accommodations, and no waiting in doctors' waiting rooms, plus valet parking. Consumers will want access, and will get it, despite the limitations of managed care networks.

U.S. consumers want choices, and they do not like to wait. The stage is being set for large-scale competition between very different approaches to healthcare delivery. Advanced Stage 4 and Stage 5 managed care markets like Albuquerque, New Mexico; Boston, Massachusetts; Los Angeles, California; Minneapolis–St. Paul, Minnesota; and Portland, Oregon will be the test kitchens for the new recipes of health reform. Most observers predict there will be only a few competing integrated systems in each regional market by the year 2000.

STRATEGIES FOR PROVIDERS, HMOs, AND SUPPLIERS

Providers

Knowing their market stage is providers' first step in building sustainable strategies for a managed care future. Then they must learn what works—and what has failed—in similar markets. Costly mistakes can be avoided via educational programs, consultants, and site visits to comparable markets that have experienced such changes. The goal is to move up the learning curve as rapidly as possible without falling off. The immediate temptation is to want to skip a stage, going directly to more sophisticated models of integration. But that will not work if physicians are not ready, if other hospitals do not yet understand the need for networking, or if HMOs are attacking aggressively instead of looking for partners. Transition strategies must be appropriate to the level of HMO market penetration. To survive, providers must plan ahead, create a shared vision (and shared risk-pool!) for cost-containing partnerships, and move into higher-stage strategies earlier than competitors.

HMOs

Managed care plans may make the mistake of attacking immature marketplaces with advanced strategies. Such moves will improve short-term profits, but will also trigger a backlash and diminish future prospects for payer-provider cooperation. Some insurers and HMOs believe the current surplus of hospitals and physician specialists is a buyer's market. Treating providers like a commodity to be exploited is good for profit margins but poisons future relationships in which provider cooperation will be needed. HMOs need to understand that their provider network *is* the HMO to patients and payers. When employers demand HEDIS data, it will be provider performance that will be measured, not the HMO. Sufficient provider resentment of HMO discounting and micromanagement will result in provider-sponsored HMOs and provider refusals to contract with the most predatory health plans. HMOs need to think cooperation now.

Suppliers

The reality of selling in very different healthcare markets is already driving suppliers quietly crazy. Every market and customer situation is different. National strategies will not work. Now is the time for suppliers to get close to the customer and know their markets. Suppliers, device makers, and pharmaceutical firms must become intimately knowledgeable about regional and statewide networks, HMO and insurer market moves, and entrepreneurial initiatives by physician management corporations and other deal-makers. It will not be enough to sell on a wholesale basis to group purchasing organizations (GPOs) such as Voluntary Hospitals of America and American Healthcare Systems. Wholesale transactions by purchasing groups' computer-driven models will reduce suppliers to commodities. Suppliers must understand that GPOs are not driving the marketplace. Purchasing decisions will be made by capitated physician groups, staff-model HMOs, and integrated health networks. Suppliers must learn to act as partners with networks, adding value through clinical paths and sharing capitation.

SOURCES

Anders, G. "Once a Hot Specialty, Anesthesiology Cools as Insurers Scale Back," *Wall Street Journal*, 17 March 1995, pp. A1, 6.

Cathcart, R. "MUSC, Columbia/HCA Union Raises Serious Public Policy Issues," *Charlestown Post and Courier*, 12 March 1995, p. 17A.

Cerne, R. 1994. "The Minnesota Model." *Hospitals and Health Networks* 68 (11): 30–32.

Chen, E. "Gingrich Calls for an Investigation of Managed Care," *Los Angeles Times*, 29 March 1995, pp. A1, 21.

Cochrane, J. D. 1996. "Market Dynamics 1995." *Integrated Healthcare Report* 4 (1): 18.

Darby, M. 1994. "Cleveland's Payers Begin Forming Networks Based on Quality of Care." *Healthcare Systems Strategy Report* 11 (12): 7, 9.

Georges, C. "Slower Growth of Health-Care Spending Is Urged by Key Republicans in Congress," *Wall Street Journal*, 29 March 1995, pp. A2, 8.

Greenberg, D. S. "Health Reform Is Happening Anyway," *Baltimore Sun*, 23 October 1994, p. B1.

Hamer, R. 1994a. "HMO Industry Report, Part II." *InterStudy Competitive Edge* 4 (1): 1–109.

———. 1994b. "Regional Market Analysis, Part III." *InterStudy Competitive Edge* 4 (1): 1–121.

———. 1996. "HMO Industry Report." *InterStudy Competitive Edge* 6 (1): 1–136.

Heimoff, S. 1996. "Rethinking Kaiser." *California Medicine* 3 (4): 21–25.

Henderson, J. A. 1994. "Integrated Healthcare Networks: The Future Is Now." *SMG Marketing Letter* 8 (4): 2–3.

Japsen, B. 1994. "Church Puts Faith in System Mergers." *Modern Healthcare* 24 (23): 32–36.

Lord, J. T. 1994. "PHO-Itis: A Disease Affecting the American Healthcare Scene." *Health System Leader* 1 (2): 29–30.

McManis, G. 1994. "Meeting the Future: CEO Summit on the New Health Care Delivery Alliance." *Hospitals & Health Networks* 68 (11): 46.

Meyer, H. 1995. "Doctors Turn to Management Companies." *AMA News*, Feb. 13, pp. 1, 25.

Rudd, T. 1994a. "Atlanta Not-for-Profits Aren't Circling the Wagons Over Columbia/HCA Deal." *Healthcare Systems Strategy Report* 11 (12): 11–12.

———. 1994b. "Less Is More With Maryland's Newest State-wide Network. *Healthcare Systems Strategy Report* 11 (12): 1, 5–6.

Sardinha, C., and T. Rudd. 1994. "Integration Trend Spells

More Competition for Managed Care." *Managed Care Outlook* 7 (11): 1–3.

Wise, D. 1994. "Houston Group Goes Against the Grain." *Business & Health* 12 (6): 61–62.

CHAPTER 2

Managed Care Outlook: High Growth and New Markets for HMOs

It's the corporatization of health care, and what's wrong with that?
Kenneth Abramowitz, Wall Street Analyst (Eckholm 1994)

THIS IS an era of health reform—a movement driven not by the government but by the market—and the managed care takeover of U.S. healthcare is well under way. By the year 2000, another 50 million to 100 million Americans will be enrolled in HMOs and similar managed care arrangements, and HMOs will be clearly established as the dominant form of health plan (see Fig. 2.1).

Figure 2.1 HMO Enrollment Growth Projections, 1990–2000

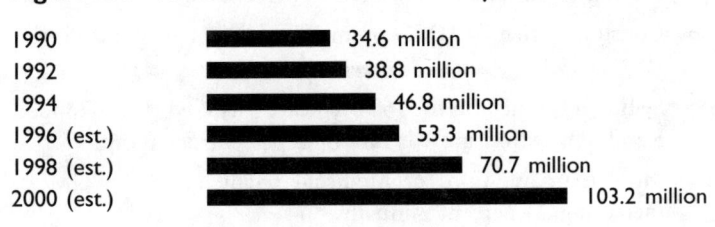

1990	34.6 million
1992	38.8 million
1994	46.8 million
1996 (est.)	53.3 million
1998 (est.)	70.7 million
2000 (est.)	103.2 million

Source: Hamer, R. 1996. "HMO Industry Report." InterStudy Competitive Edge. InterStudy Publications, Bloomington, MN.

Five Stages of Managed Care

If the HMO movement is ultimately to succeed, HMOs must satisfy consumer concerns about choice, access, and quality. In California, two consumer-led ballot initiatives aim to impose new controls over HMO management and marketing practices. Sponsors of competing versions of the California Patient Protection Act filed 1.5 million signatures to impose sweeping restrictions on managed care plans (Schine and Hammonds 1996). At least 30 other states passed managed care reform legislation in the mid-1990s, such as mandatory two-day hospital stays for newborns. Federal legislation on the 48-hour stay was enacted in the fall of 1996, shortly before the national election. HMOs must move quickly to satisfy consumer concerns or there will be more government regulation of the managed care industry.

HIGH GROWTH AND NEW MARKETS FOR HMOs

HMO enrollment is climbing, and not just in the West. Industry observers see HMO penetration reaching 50 percent in the Mid-Atlantic and South Central regions by the year 2000 (Schachner 1996). Major metropolitan areas like Atlanta, Boston, Chicago, Dallas, and Denver have as many as 20 HMOs competing aggressively on price.

Employers, seniors, and Medicaid recipients are signing up with health maintenance organizations in record numbers. By the end of this decade, some 40 percent of all Americans may belong to HMOs. At that point, 65 to 70 percent of the commercial (employer-sponsored, under age 65) lives may belong to HMOs, as well as 20 to 25 percent of Medicare eligibles and 60 to 65 percent of Medicaid recipients. Growth statistics from InterStudy show the pattern of HMOs' national growth:

- Combined pure and point-of-service HMO enrollment is soaring at an annual rate of 12.9 percent.
- Consumer-friendly HMO point-of-service plans grew 56 percent in 1995.
- Senior enrollment in the 168 Medicare-qualified HMOs topped 5 million, with a growth rate of 2 percent per month.
- More than one-third of Medicaid recipients are in HMOs, increasing 23 percent annually.
- California, Pennsylvania, New York, Florida, and Oregon had a combined HMO enrollment boost of 2.9 million in 1994. (Hamer 1996)

UNITED STATES NEARS FINAL STAGE OF MANAGED CARE TAKEOVER

In the remaining years of the 1990s, U.S. health insurers will convert the last remaining enrollees of indemnity insurance into managed care alternatives, especially HMOs and point-of-service plans. This will be a private-sector development, as employers shift their employees and retirees into lower-cost HMO options. Government-sponsored beneficiaries—Medicare and Medicaid—will be converted wholesale to at-risk HMO plans.

Highlights of this dramatic transformation to managed care include:

- Two out of three insured Americans are enrolled in HMOs and managed care plans, according to a study of companies with more than 200 employees by KPMG–Peat Marwick.
- For-profit HMOs now enroll more members than nonprofit plans like Kaiser, HIP of New York, and Seattle-based Group Health of Puget Sound.
- Three-fourths of all physicians have signed contracts with HMOs and managed care plans; 89 percent of doctors employed in group practices are working under managed care agreements.
- All 50 states have HMOs; Alaska and Wyoming were the last to develop HMO plans. (Eckholm 1994)

The rapid growth of HMOs and private-sector healthcare has been little noticed since the Clinton election. In 1993, the year that Hillary Clinton drew headlines fighting Congress for universal health coverage, the health field was swept by $20 billion of mergers and acquisitions involving hospitals, physicians, medical laboratories, long-term care and rehabilitation facilities, and medical supplies, up from $6 billion in 1992. Now that fears of a government takeover of healthcare are easing, the nation's $1 trillion health industry is positioned for market-led reforms to control healthcare costs and cut utilization to record lows.

The privatization of healthcare has drawn praise from market-minded conservatives, who note that the medical care component of the consumer price index (CPI) rose only 7 percent in 1994. But the increasing power of HMOs and managed care programs draws criticism from worried health professionals like Dr. Arnold Relman, editor emeritus of the *New England Journal of Medicine*, who protests, "There's never been a time in the history of American medicine when the independence and autonomy of American medical practitioners was as uncertain as it is now" (Eckholm 1994).

TOP 10 TRENDS FOR MANAGED CARE TO THE YEAR 2000

These will be the top 10 trends for HMOs and managed care to the year 2000.

Trend 1. Enrollment Gain

A majority of Americans will rely on HMOs to provide their health coverage and medical services. HMOs experienced double-digit growth in 1994, climbing past the 50 million enrollment mark on a national basis with an 11.5 percent increase (Sardinha 1994a). The gain of 5.3 million new enrollees is the biggest HMO membership gain in a single year since the Group Health Association of America (GHAA) started keeping enrollment statistics in 1988. The next five years will experience accelerating rates for conversion of PPOs and managed indemnity plans to the HMO model.

The most important factor in the shift to HMOs is the growing preference of employers for managed care. In 1991, only 47 percent of company-sponsored enrollees were in HMOs, soaring to 65 percent by 1994 (Eckholm 1994). Employers are now showing their preference for HMOs, and their competitive prices, over traditional health plans that offer more consumer choice but are often priced 15 to 25 percent higher.

Now that HMOs have convinced employers to try managed care, can HMOs satisfy customer demands for quality service? HMOs must face the business challenge to win consumers with price but hold them with service. Can HMOs keep their enrollees satisfied despite limits on physician access and denying "unnecessary" services that consumers want anyway? HMOs are now stressing their commitment to quality, and producing report cards that analyze clinical outcomes and customer satisfaction.

Trend 2. Medicaid Capitation

State-level Medicaid reform is now the principal focus of government-sponsored reform efforts. The Health Care Financing Administration (HCFA) has approved eight waivers to allow states to pursue managed-care reform initiatives, and seven more states are seeking HCFA approvals. The growing number of state waiver requests has caused the federal Physician Payment Review Commission to question whether the HCFA waiver program has been stretched too far and should be expanded or modified (Gardner 1994).

Medicaid HMO enrollment boomed by 63 percent in 1994 (Kertesz 1994). States are shifting Medicaid beneficiaries into managed care plans at a rapid rate. The Department of Health and Human Services reported an increase of three million enrollees in the number of Medicaid patients signed up with HMOs and managed care programs. At the end of 1994, some 7.8 million of the nation's 31.2 million Medicaid eligibles were HMO members, up from 4.8 million in 1993. As of 1994, managed care plans served Medicaid patients in 44 states, and 38 percent of HMOs in a survey had plans to get into Medicaid risk contracting in 1995 (Sardinha 1994a).

The most common types of Medicaid managed care programs are: (1) capitation to provide all or part of the Medicaid benefits on a prepaid risk basis; and (2) primary care case-management programs, in which physicians contract with the state to provide primary care and gatekeeper services, coordinating referrals to specialists and hospitals.

State governors and legislatures are no longer waiting for Washington to solve their Medicaid costs issues. The momentum for government-sponsored reform efforts is now coming from the states. Over 50 percent of the big increase in Medicaid managed care has been driven by state health reform initiatives in states like Oregon, Tennessee, Kentucky, and California. Governors have put their weight behind the shift to managed care to control soaring state-level expenditures for Medicaid. More than 1.6 million of the new Medicaid enrollees joined under health reform demonstration projects, which expand eligibility but put limits on costs.

Trend 3. Medicare HMOs

Providers must take notice of the fact that Medicare beneficiaries are switching to HMOs at increasing rates. An estimated 7 percent, or 2.2 million of the 33 million Medicare eligibles, had signed up with HMOs by the end of 1995—double the number signed up in 1989—and many more are expected to switch (Eckholm 1995). Heavily penetrated HMO markets like Southern California, Oregon, and Minnesota have 25 to 50 percent of Medicare patients enrolled in managed care plans.

HCFA's guidelines on Medicare point-of-service plans were released in November 1994. Under the POS rules, only 10 percent of an HMO POS plan's medical expenses can be for out-of-network care. The POS option is likely to appeal to Medicare patients who want to keep a physician relationship but are attracted by the HMO's low copayments (typically $5 per visit) and drug benefits, which may range from $500 to $1,200 per year.

HMOs are targeting the Medicare market, especially in high-cost regions where Medicare HMO payments are higher, even with the federal government's 95 percent payment formula. Some 38 percent of HMOs offered a Medicare product in 1995, compared with only 7 percent in 1994 (Sardinha 1994a). A controversy over the funding formula could slow HMO entrance into the Medicare market. Federal officials are studying ways to adjust Medicare HMO payments to account for the fact that HMOs "skim off the cream" of the healthiest patients in each market, leaving older, sicker seniors in the pool whose costs are used to establish HMO prices.

Medicare beneficiaries seem to like managed care. Rita Schlageter, a senior citizen from Mineola, New York, enrolled with the Oxford HMO and used the cost savings "to play more golf and stuff" (Eckholm 1995). Recent Medicare HMO enrollees are especially satisfied with their managed care plans when their physician is a member of the HMO panel. Twice as many Medicare beneficiaries enrolled in an HMO than disenrolled in 1993, according to the federal Prospective Payment Assessment Commission (Fortuna 1994). Medicare patients seemed to prefer staff- and group-model HMOs, like the Kaiser plan or HIP of New York, to independent practice associations. This may reflect the fact that some of the enrollees may already have been long-time enrollees with the HMO before becoming Medicare-eligible.

The Republican majority elected to Congress in 1994 believes HMOs could be key to reducing Medicare and Medicaid costs. Encouraging Medicare's conversion to managed care could be a major factor in federal budget deficit reduction in the next few years. Immediately after taking power in January 1995, congressional GOP leader Newt Gingrich suggested that the Medicare insurance program ought to be replaced with a more efficient and less government-directed system, like private health maintenance organizations, to reduce Medicare's $160 billion cost (Wines 1995).

Medicare HMOs may be a beneficiary of the new GOP majority's pledge to balance the federal budget within five to seven years. Medicare budget cuts of $223 billion would be required over seven years, and Medicaid cuts of $268 billion, according to budget estimates by Tim Muris, a former Reagan Administration official who specializes in health costs (*Los Angeles Times* 1994). The potential reductions in federal health spending would be twice as deep as the Clinton health proposal of 1994. Drastic cuts in Medicare funding would force individuals to pay much more for their health in copayments and deductibles—or drive many Medicare eligibles to join HMOs and other managed care networks.

Medicare outlays could rise to $286 billion annually by the year 2000. Because HMOs are paid only 95 percent of actual Medicare costs, the federal government could lower its Medicare outlays by

5 percent, or $14.3 billion, if all Medicare beneficiaries signed up with HMOs. Even more savings might be possible in the future if Republican conservatives put the entire Medicare program out to bid, letting HMOs and insurers compete with no price guarantees. HCFA officials could take their cues from private employers, who are gaining price concessions from HMOs and actually lowering their health costs.

Trend 4. Price Wars

Competition among health insurers and aggressive negotiating by major employers are driving down HMO premiums and prices. According to GHAA, HMO premiums were down 1.2 percent in 1995, following increases of 5.6 percent in 1994 and 8.1 percent in 1993. The upside of HMO competition has been lower inflation on a national basis. Health inflation, the medical care component of the CPI, was only 4.9 percent by years' end in 1994, as the overall consumer price index held at a modest 2.7 percent annual increase (Hershey 1995).

The HMO price war is the result of "increased competition among HMOs, increased competition among physicians and hospitals, and increased price sensitivity on the part of consumers," according to GHAA director of research Jon Gabel, when the data were released in Washington, D.C. (Sardinha 1994a). The result has been lower prices for HMO stocks like United Healthcare, U.S. Healthcare, PacifiCare, and FHP, many of which lost 10 to 15 percent of share price in late 1994 as Wall Street analysts figured the effect of price cuts on 1995 earnings. Still, HMOs are the best long-term investment in a restructured healthcare market.

The new data suggest that HMO prices are not immune to the "six-year insurance cycle," the long-term tendency of insurance to rise and fall in a predictable pattern. HMO profits rose from 1991 through 1993 but began to erode in 1994 and worsened in 1995. Some employers are demanding steeper rate cuts. After three years of price increases in central Massachusetts, a wave of price competition swept the state's larger HMOs: The average HMO premium rose only 1.5 percent for large employer groups and less than 1 percent for small groups, according to a study by the Massachusetts Rate Setting Commission (Cochrane 1994).

Price wars have boosted HMO enrollments, but at the cost of declining profits. Princeton health economist Dr. Uwe Reinhardt observes, "It was absolutely predictable that those margins would be competed away until they were paper thin" (McGuire 1996, 1). Deep provider discounts are helping sustain HMO profits, but the "predatory pricing" of some HMOs to buy marketshare may be

Five Stages of Managed Care

winding down. A warning signal about HMO prices came from the trend-setting California marketplace. The Pacific Business Group on Health, an employer coalition in the San Francisco Bay Area, and the California Public Employees Retirement System (CalPERS) faced price hikes of only 1 to 2 percent from PacifiCare and FHP, 2 of its 17 managed care plans (Marsh 1996). The state-sponsored health insurance plan that serves 112,000 small-business employees held rates flat after cuts of 15 percent in 1993, 6.2 percent in 1994, and 5 percent in 1995.

Trend 5. Capitation

The conversion of providers to capitation-based payment may be one of the most important—and controversial—HMO strategies of the 1990s. Sharing up to 80 percent of the HMO premium with providers creates new incentives for cost reductions to HMOs. Capitated providers can keep the savings of reducing hospital use, diagnostic procedures, and unnecessary surgeries. The early results from capitating providers have been astonishing. Providers have slashed utilization rates for some services by as much as 60 percent and more (see Table 2.1).

Provider capitation is the most successful strategy HMOs have ever employed for drastically lowering health costs and use rates. The incentives of capitation are fundamentally the reverse of traditional fee-for-service. Under capitation, providers are rewarded

Table 2.1
Utilization of Services May Drop 15 to 60 Percent Under Capitation

Service	Unmanaged Rate*	Moderately Managed Rate*	Percentage Decline
Hospital component			
Inpatient days	430	260	40%
Radiology	375	145	61%
Laboratory (outpatient)	500	220	56%
Professional component			
Surgery	1,540	800	48%
Radiology	1,250	820	34%
Diagnostic testing	480	250	50%
Office visits	3,300	2,900	12%

*Utilization rate per 1,000 commercial non-Medicare enrollees.
Source: Estimates by BDC Advisors, San Francisco; cited in "Capitation Strategies," Advisory Board Company, Washington, D.C., 1994, p. 11.

for doing less rather than more. Utilization drops, often overnight, after providers sign capitation agreements. Physicians practice a new kind of cost-cutting medicine. Clinical efficiency—not revenue maximization by providing more services—is the standard by which physicians practice when capitated.

The question for the next few years is: Will HMOs shift providers to capitation? Or will HMOs prefer to remain in control, by micromanaging physician and hospital use while paying providers discounted fees and per diem payments? HMOs on the West Coast have been more accepting of provider capitation, but East Coast HMOs have been slower to turn control over to providers. Big HMOs like U.S. Healthcare and United Healthcare prefer to micromanage providers, and keep doctors and hospitals on discounted fee schedules and per diem payments. Lack of organized physician groups in the East and South has slowed the spread of capitation in those markets.

Some HMOs are purchasing physician practices and developing HMO-owned primary care networks as an alternative to capitation. The HMOs remain in full control, as their captive gatekeepers limit access to specialists and hospitals. In California, Foundation Health Plan announced it would spend $120 million to construct a statewide network of 26 staff-model clinics throughout California (Cochrane 1994). All of the Foundation physicians would be capitated, with their incentives aligned with the HMO. Foundation recruited or acquired 76 physicians, and planned to double its medical organization, but has more recently backed away from such aggressive physician acquisition. Foundation's change of strategy may have been influenced by rival FHP, an HMO based in Long Beach, California, to spin off its 400-doctor medical group into an independent unit.

Doctors and hospitals building PHOs will find insurers competing for physician loyalty in the next few years. National insurers like Aetna, Prudential, and Blue Cross are spending millions on building physician networks. New York Life Insurance, through its Sanus Health Systems subsidiary, has purchased 13 practices in New York and Long Island. Similiar plans to build insurer-owned networks are proceeding in New Jersey, where Blue Cross and Blue Shield opened 10 health centers in 1995 (Miller 1994b).

Trend 6. Point-of-Service Plans

The popularity of point-of-service plans continues to grow. About 5 million HMO members were enrolled in POS plans in 1995, an increase of 56 percent from 1994, according to a report by

Five Stages of Managed Care

InterStudy (Hamer 1996). Almost two out of three HMOs offer POS options (see Fig. 2.2), which could climb to 75 percent, according to a report by the Group Health Association of America (1994). In markets like New England and the Mid-Atlantic, POS plans are more popular than traditional "pure" HMOs (Hamer 1996).

The POS plan is the fastest-growing HMO type in the nation. Most (9 out of 10) new POS enrollees joined large plans with more than 25,000 enrollees. Over 300 plans, 60 percent of all HMOs, offer a POS product. Many more HMOs are scrambling to offer the open-network option to convert "pure" (closed-panel) HMO members, who will pay a little more for choice, as well as PPO enrollees, who will save money by switching to HMO point-of-service plans. This option has the strongest appeal in the Northeast and Mid-Atlantic states. Almost 600,000 POS members signed up in the Mid-Atlantic region (New Jersey, New York, and Pennsylvania). Blue Cross/Blue Shield plans were leaders in the aggressive marketing of POS plans. In 1995, more than half (56 percent) of all Blues plans offered POS options, and with an average POS enrollment of over 10,000 per plan (Hamer 1996).

Trend 7. Blues Mergers

America's Blue Cross and Blue Shield plans are coming together to battle national insurers and independent HMO plans through mergers, strategic affiliations, and joint ventures. In the next few years, the number of Blues plans could shrink by 25 to 35 percent, and the number of multistate plans could grow to 10, 15, or more. The consolidation trend among the Blues parallels the merger trend among independent HMOs. Newly merged, larger HMOs

Figure 2.2 HMOs Offering Point-of-Service or Open-Ended Products, 1991–95

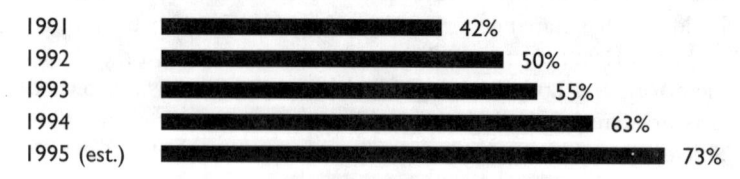

Year	Percentage
1991	42%
1992	50%
1993	55%
1994	63%
1995 (est.)	73%

Source: Group Health Association of America. 1994. National Directory of HMOs Database; cited in Sardinha, C. 1994. "Media Blitz Helps U.S. Healthcare Make Inroads in Atlanta." Managed Care Outlook 7 (24): 1.

plan to slash their administrative costs and offer comparable plans in multiple states.

Blues mergers are breaking out from the Midwest to the far West. Two midwestern Blues plans—Community Mutual Insurance of Cincinnati and the Associated Group of Indianapolis—merged in 1996 to produce Anthem, a new company with more than 7 million enrollees and $5 billion in assets. The deal created the fourth-largest Blues plan in the nation, operating in Kentucky, Indiana, and Ohio. Anthem may become the nation's second-largest Blues organization, after completing a merger with Blue Cross and Blue Shield of New Jersey, thus adding another 1.9 million subscribers (Freudenheim 1996). The combined company would have combined revenues of $9 billion. The story is the same in the Northwest: Blue Cross of Washington and Alaska, in Seattle, and the Medical Service Corporation of Eastern Washington, in Spokane, have merged to form PREMERA, which serves more than 1 million Blue Cross customers in Alaska, Oregon, and Washington.

Eleven Blues plans created in 1994 a National Accounts Consortium to serve large employers that operate in multiple states. The joint venture improves the Blues' ability to compete with national insurers like Aetna, Cigna, and Prudential for Fortune 500 companies. The Blues plans streamlined such functions as service delivery, network credentialing, data reporting, customer service, and medical policies.

Trend 8. HMO-PPO Blurring Boundaries

Within the next few years, the distinctions between HMOs and PPOs will have all but disappeared. Market forces and state regulations are driving PPOs to assume financial risk and manage costs and utilization like HMOs. In Washington, Ethix Northwest Seattle, with 175,000 PPO enrollees, received a state license as a health services contractor, which allows the plan to assume risk under Washington's health reform statute (Sardinha 1994b). Ethix's market strategy is to team up with hospitals and physicians to create local HMOs, with provider risk-sharing. The concept of small HMOs built on local physician-hospital organizations flies in the face of conventional industry wisdom that only very large, vertically-integrated HMOs can survive.

In Minneapolis, a hotbed of managed care activity, Preferred One is converting PPO enrollees into risk products with capitation. Preferred One is in discussions with four insurers to create new models for risk-bearing. Under Minnesota's health reform statute,

Five Stages of Managed Care

scheduled for implementation in July 1997, all health plans in the state must become risk-assuming entities. In the transition process, Preferred One will run a fee-for-service network alongside the capitated network. Not all Minnesota providers want capitation, and many employers are not ready to convert their self-funded health plans to full risk.

Trend 9. Consolidation

Consolidations, mergers, and acquisitions will accelerate over the rest of the decade. Big HMOs and insurers will get bigger to:

- increase marketshare;
- dominate markets;
- eliminate smaller competitors;
- reduce price competition;
- increase leverage with providers;
- promote brand-name recognition;
- price products more competitively;
- reduce administrative costs;
- share information systems;
- develop systems and protocols to manage risk and utilization;
- produce more comprehensive report cards for purchasers;
- pool capital; and
- invest in staff-model delivery systems.

A number of health plans are sitting on huge cash reserves, including Minnesota's United Healthcare, California's Wellpoint, and a number of local Blue Cross plans.

The mega-merger of Aetna and U.S. Healthcare created the nation's largest managed care organization, with a combined enrollment of 10.3 million and revenues of $16,587.7 million, according to Aetna. In 1994, Metropolitan and the Travelers agreed to align the healthcare facets of their business. Even combined, however, Metropolitan and the Travelers did not like the prospects of the managed care market, and sold their MetraHealth business to United Healthcare in 1996. Prudential may follow a similar strategy, according to speculation in the *New York Times* (Quint 1995).

Mergers and consolidations would drive down administrative costs and create economies of scale. The biggest HMOs and insurers are fighting to slash overhead to turn a $100 million to $200 million pool of "unnecessary costs" into potential profits (Loomis 1994).

Combining health insurers would slash overhead and improve profits. Now that managed care controls more than half of the health insurance market, the conversion of much of the rest of the traditional indemnity and government-sponsored health plans is moving at a brisk pace. Many of the top 20 health plans are independent HMOs, and the large commercial insurers and Blues plans are rapidly converting their enrollees to managed care (see Table 2.2).

The best rationale for consolidation may not be marketshare but economies of scale in administrative costs. Larger HMOs have significantly lower administrative costs—only one-third of

Table 2.2
Top 20 U.S. Health Plans

Company and Location	Type	1993 Revenues (in millions)
Kaiser Permanente, Oakland, California	HMO	$9,728
Prudential of America, Newark, New Jersey	Commercial	8,600
BC/BS of Michigan, Detroit, Michigan	Blue	6,248
Empire BC/BS, New York	Blue	5,388
Cigna, Philadelphia, Pennsylvania	Commercial	5,384
Aetna, Hartford, Connecticut	Commercial	4,494
BC/BS of Massachusetts, Boston	Blue	3,753
Principal Financial Group, Des Moines, Iowa	Commercial	3,417
Health Care Service, Chicago, Illinois	Blue	3,399
FHP International, California	HMO	3,250
Humana, Louisville, Kentucky	HMO	3,147
Metropolitan Life, New York	Commercial	2,997
BC of California/Wellpoint, Los Angeles, California	HMO	2,896
Travelers, Hartford, Connecticut	Commercial	2,686
U.S. Healthcare, Pennsylvania	HMO	2,625
Guardian, New York	Commercial	2,555
United Healthcare, Minnesota	HMO	2,469
Community Mutual, Cincinnati, Ohio	Blue	2,270
BC/BS of Virginia, Richmond, Virginia	Blue	2,210
Mutual of Omaha, Nebraska	Commercial	2,126

Source: FORTUNE © 1994 Time, Inc. All rights reserved.

smaller plans, according to the annual industry profile compiled by the GHAA (1994). HMOs with more than 250,000 members achieve real economies of scale in managing their products. Size is no guarantee of profitability, however. Large plans of 250,000-plus enrollees had somewhat lower profits, at 2.6 percent, than midsized plans of 100,000 to 250,000 members, with net margins of 3.4 percent in 1994. Larger plans tend to have greater numbers of older enrollees, with higher costs of care, explaining the profit difference.

Trend 10. Provider-Sponsored Plans

Healthcare providers in Stage 2 and Stage 3 markets are entering the market with their own HMOs and managed care products. There were 131 provider-sponsored HMOs at the end of 1995, according to InterStudy, with a combined enrollment of more than 5 million covered lives, about 10 percent of all HMO enrollees (Hamer 1996). Providers are building, buying, and forming joint-venture HMOs with established insurers. The goal is to build a fully integrated delivery network that includes the financing as well as delivery components. Providers are becoming aware of the profit potential in owning their own HMOs, too. If the HMO is making the most money in the food chain of capitation and managed care, then providers should own HMOs, moving upstream in the dollar flow.

In the Northwest, hospitals and physicians are investing millions to build HMOs. The Washington market already includes successful provider-sponsored managed care plans, including an HMO and a PPO owned by the Seattle-based Sisters of Providence. Now Swedish Health Services of Seattle and Tacoma-based MultiCare Health System have purchased a 3,000-member HMO from Cigna. Next is coming UnifiedPhysicians of Washington, a spinoff of the state medical association. The doctors raised nearly $6 million to start a statewide HMO (Miller 1994a).

More physician-sponsored HMOs are emerging. According to a study by Towers Perrin, 38 of the nation's 50 state medical societies are planning or actively developing managed care plans (Miller 1994b). Two state societies are already operating HMOs, and three more physician associations have PPOs. In California, the California Medical Association's California Advantage plan has the backing of 6,700 physician investors, with planned growth to 10,000 of California's 75,000 doctors. Some 30,000 California physicians participate in the state association's provider network, whose strategy is to enter the market as a PPO, with an insurance partnership to provide a full-risk product, ultimately including capitated Medicaid and Medicare.

The move to physician-sponsored HMOs is controversial in some states. Colorado physicians rejected a state society plan to levy $100 from every member for an HMO feasibility project. The Kansas Medical Society, on the other hand, raised nearly $5 million in startup capital to create Heartland Health Systems, going operational as an HMO in 1995.

Physician-hospital networks are using their seller's clout to create managed care joint venturers with insurers. In Chicago, Rush–Presbyterian–St. Luke's Medical Center entered into a fifty-fifty joint venture with Prudential (Cerne 1994). The arrangement merged the operations of Rush's Anchor HMO, a 115,000-enrollee staff-model HMO, with Prudential's 83,000-enrollee network-model HMO and a point-of-service plan with 157,000 members. In response, Northwestern Health Network, a nine-hospital affiliated system anchored by Northwestern Memorial Hospital in downtown Chicago, is negotiating with United Healthcare to create a network of physician clinics. Consolidation is accelerating in Chicago, where Aetna Plans has established six physician-operated clinics, and Humana expanded its 22 staff-model HMO clinics with 62 affiliated physician groups and 11 capitated hospitals. Providers and HMOs are jockeying to dominate twenty-first century healthcare.

THE FUTURE OF HMOs AND PROVIDERS: COMPETE OR CONSOLIDATE?

The biggest question in any forecast of HMO futures is: Will HMOs compete or consolidate with their provider networks? The last push to control the nation's $1 trillion health industry is beginning, and it will be a billion-dollar battle of consolidation, acquisition, and price warfare. HMOs and insurers want to dominate healthcare. Providers are fighting back with their own managed care plans. There are too few instances of collaboration like Allina in Minnesota, the merger of an HMO and a regional provider network.

Looking to a managed care–dominated future, there are a range of options for HMOs, insurers, and providers:

- *Competition* is the most likely strategy for both HMOs and insurers, as the health plans confront at-risk provider networks by refusing to share capitation, micromanaging provider performance, exploiting surplus capacity with low-ball prices, and dumping providers if they complain.
- HMOs can create their own staff-model organizations by *purchasing providers*, beginning with primary care physicians,

and acquiring specialists and hospitals as enrollment rises to appropriate volume levels.
- HMOs and insurers can acquire primary care physicians but "rent" specialists and hospitals on a partial fee-for-service and per diem basis, to control health plans via *partial integration*.
- HMOs and provider networks can form *joint ventures*, sharing ownership in twenty-eighty to fifty-fifty equity arrangements. (Most joint ventures today are dominated by HMOs or insurers.)
- *Providers can invest* in HMO plans and products to promote physician and hospital commitment to cost management.
- Providers can sponsor HMOs to compete head-to-head with established HMOs and insurers.

Providers are moving aggressively toward integration. A national survey by Deloitte & Touche found 88 percent of hospitals and 69 percent of physicians deeply involved in integration activities and only 55 percent of managed care organizations with integration plans (Shriver 1994). Providers have to move in this direction. Hospitals and doctors lack the four components essential for success in a capitation–managed care market, the tools and systems for managing: (1) networks, (2) risk, (3) quality, and (4) information.

Forces for integrating health plans and providers are growing. Minnesota-based Allina resulted from a merger of Medica, the region's number-two HMO, and HealthSpan, a large hub-and-spoke health system. Allina coexecutive Gordon Springer claims: "The market is saying, 'We aren't going to tolerate this fragmented delivery system'" (Shriver 1994). The message is being heard. In southern Arizona, Tucson Medical Center, a regional healthcare delivery system, merged with the Partners Health Plan, a regional HMO with 110,000 enrollees (Burns 1994). Two physician IPAs will also join the integrated system, to be called HealthPartners Health Plan. Together, the merged plan will serve 200,000 enrollees, with joint revenues of $400 million.

LOOKING FORWARD: PARTNERSHIP IS THE ONLY WIN-WIN STRATEGY

For health systems to become fully integrated in a partnership models will not be easy. It will require overcoming competitive attitudes between HMOs and providers and smoothing over almost 20 years of hard bargaining and payer-driven discounts. In some markets, providers and overaggressive HMOs continue to war over the plans' predatory tactics and bottom-level prices. Simply organizing provider networks to prevent managed care discounts will not work. Eight New York hospitals were forced to disband their regional network after a Justice Department investigation of the network's attempt to limit HMO discounts to 10 percent (Pallarito 1994).

In Atlanta, U.S. Healthcare is running head-on into provider resistance. To enter the Atlanta marketplace, the HMO is spending millions to move into Georgia but is struggling to overcome hostility from doctors and hospitals over U.S. Healthcare's tough negotiating tactics and "very, very aggressive rates." An Atlanta hospital executive characterizes U.S. Healthcare's contracting approach as "a cookbook," adding that his hospital would not contract with the plan even though U.S. Healthcare now is "coming up with rates higher than what we proposed a year ago" (Sardinha 1994c).

Ultimately, competition between managed care plans and providers will not work. The market will force them together. A reasonable first goal would be for them to integrate such functions as utilization review, cost management, provider credentialing, quality assurance, customer service, and information systems.

Cooperation could save all parties a lot of money, beginning with the estimated 15 to 25 percent administrative cost of managing U.S. healthcare. With cooperation, a truly integrated delivery system–HMO could eliminate 8 to 15 percent of its costs, or more. Reducing costs and satisfying customers must be the shared goals of America's 600 HMOs and 5,000 community hospitals. Integration is the only win-win strategy. All tactics that rely on competition are win-lose or lose-lose.

STRATEGIES FOR PROVIDERS, HMOs, AND SUPPLIERS

Providers

Providers' first step toward developing a managed care strategy is to recognize that managed care's takeover is inevitable. Then they must move swiftly to organize. Hospitals have generally taken the lead in restructuring for managed care, creating PHOs with those doctors who are ready to join. Physicians may resent what they consider moves by hospitals to dominate any future relationship, and some doctors are forming independent physician organizations. Perhaps the best equation for the future is:

PO (Physician Organization) + HO (Hospital Organization) = PHO.

HMOs

Traditional health insurance is dead in the mass market. Some open-choice plans may survive into the twenty-first century, as premium-priced options in corporate "cafeteria" benefit plans. Indemnity health carriers are converting rapidly to HMO models, with most offering a point-of-service option. There is a window of opportunity for marketing new HMOs in many Stage 1 through Stage 3 markets. Providers thinking about HMO development will respond positively to HMOs that offer joint ventures. HMOs that fail to seek provider partnerships may find themselves reduced to providing administrative-services-only support to at-risk provider networks that are dealing directly with employers and business coalitions in sophisticated Stage 4 and Stage 5 markets. Sophisticated purchasers will not tolerate for long HMOs that spend less than 70 percent of revenues on medical care.

Suppliers

The massive growth of HMOs is a threat and an opportunity for healthcare suppliers. They must recognize the threat. Utilization of many drugs, devices, types of equipment, and consumables will fall just as quickly as patient days and procedures. The 1990s are a watershed time for healthcare suppliers; the high points for sales and profits are all disappearing into the past. The battle for marketshare is well engaged, and consolidation is already widespread. Suppliers who fail to grasp how quickly this market transformation will occur, and who employ strategies of prudence and caution, will be rewarded by market isolation and obsolescence. The time to pull out all the stops is now.

SOURCES

Burns, J. 1994. "Arizona Providers Form Statewide Network." *Modern Healthcare* 24 (50): 20.

Cerne, F. 1994. "Chicago: Market Evolution Gains Momentum in the Windy City." *Hospitals & Health Networks* 68 (24): 48–52.

Cochrane, J. 1994. "November Quakes in Northern California." *Integrated Healthcare Report* (November): 9–12.

Eckholm, E. "While Congress Remains Silent, Health Care Transforms Itself," *New York Times*, 18 December 1994, pp. A1, 22.

———. "HMOs Are Changing the Face of Medicare," *New York Times*, 11 January 1995, pp. A1, 16.

Fortuna, G. 1994. "More Medicare Beneficiaries Are Happy with Their HMOs." *Managed Care Outlook* 7 (24): 8.

Freudenheim, J. "Health Plans In New Jersey: Blue Cross–Anthem Deal Will Create New Giant," *New York Times*, 30 May 1996, pp. C1, C4.

Gardner, J. 1994. "PPRC Debates Differing Changes in Growing State Waiver Program." *Modern Healthcare* 24 (51): 21.

Group Health Association of America. 1994. *HMO Industry Profile: 1994 Annual Edition.* Washington, DC: The Association.

Hamer, R. 1996. "HMO Industry Report." *InterStudy Competitive Edge* 6 (1): 1–136.

Hershey, R. D. "Another Year of Little Rise in Inflation," *New York Times*, 12 January 1995, pp. C1, 15.

Kertesz, L. 1995. "A Jump in Medicaid Managed Care." *Modern Healthcare* 24 (51): 21.

Loomis, C. 1994. "The Real Action in Health Care." *Fortune* (July): 149–57.

Los Angeles Times. "Republicans Told They Must Slash Medicare, Report Says," 8 January 1994, p. A13.

Marsh, B. "HMO Premiums Are Heading Higher for California Workers," *Los Angeles Times*, 30 July 1996, pp. D1, D15.

McGuire, D. 1996. "Falling Managed Care Margins Not the Result of Price Gouging." *Managed Care Outlook* 9 (14): 1–2.

Miller, J. 1994a. "New York City Insurers on the Practice Acquisition Trail." *Integrated Healthcare Report* 3 (11): 13.

———. 1994b. "Washington State Systems Buy HMO from Cigna; Washington State Medical Association to Start HMO." *Integrated Healthcare Report* 3 (11): 13.

Pallarito, K. 1994. "Justice Department Settles Eight-Hospital Case in New York." *Modern Healthcare* 24 (50): 10.

Quint, M. "Prudential Insurance May Face Specter of Losses," *New York Times*, 12 January 1995, pp. C1, 14.

Sardinha, C. 1994a. "Competition, Employer Clout Push HMO Premiums Down 1.2%." *Managed Care Outlook* 7 (24): 5.

———. 1994b. "Market Forces, State Regs Drive PPOs to Assume More Risks." *Managed Care Outlook* 7 (24): 9.

———. 1994c. "Media Blitz Helps U.S. Healthcare Make Inroads in Atlanta Market." *Managed Care Outlook* 7 (24): 1–3.

Schachner, M. 1996. "HMO Enrollment Picking Up Speed." *Business Insurance* (March): 6.

Schine, E., and K. H. Hammonds. 1996. "Hell No, HMO!" *Business Week* May 20, p. 36.

Shriver, K. 1994. "Study: Most Hospitals Will Try Integration Despite Obstacles." *Hospitals & Health Networks* 24 (50): 4.

Wines, M. "Democrats Assail GOP on Budget," *New York Times*, 7 January 1995, pp. A1, 8.

CHAPTER 3

Capitation: A New Balance of Power for HMOs and Providers

Capitation is the way of the world. Providers have to accept it as a given.
Paul Reeb, M.D., Sharp Community Medical Group, San Diego, California (Advisory Board Company 1994)

CAPITATION WILL shortly become the dominant form of payment in U.S. healthcare delivery. Under capitated contracts, HMOs and insurers pay physicians and hospitals a fixed amount per month for each health plan member, regardless of whether a member makes 20 visits, has open heart surgery, or never sets foot through the providers' doors (Mayer 1994). Replacing fee-for-service payments to doctors and per diem payments to hospitals, capitation is a per capita budget for a managed care market.

The shift to capitation is the most important change in healthcare financing since the advent of prospective payment systems and Medicare's adoption of diagnosis-related groups. It is a revolution in healthcare reimbursement for payers and providers, because it is fundamentally restructuring healthcare delivery, not just payment patterns.

Why is capitation replacing other payment arrangements?

- Purchasers—HMOs, insurers, governments, or employers—can shift 100 percent of their financial risk to providers.
- Purchasers know exactly how much their healthcare services and benefits cost.

Five Stages of Managed Care

- Providers regain control of all monies for patient care.
- Distribution of healthcare services and payments comes under provider control.
- Purchasers can reduce their administrative overhead costs, because providers take on responsibility for utilization management and quality assurance.
- Consumers know that all services are covered.
- Consumers can identify a primary physician to coordinate all their care needs.

Capitation is supplying the incentives for integration that the U.S. healthcare industry has badly needed. Today's pluralistic system is based on payments that fragment care. Traditional fee-for-service reimbursement has created separate industries—hospitals, physician care, long-term care. As HMOs and insurers convert to capitation, however, providers assume the position of insurer—they become both risk holder and risk manager.

PAYERS AND PROVIDERS SHARE RISKS AND REWARDS

Many providers welcome capitation because, through this form of reimbursement, *they regain control of dollars and patients*. The arrangement is simple: Providers accept a fixed-sum payment to provide all healthcare services. If physicians and hospitals are clinically efficient and keep the costs of care below their capitation payment, they make money. If not, they lose money.

On the West Coast, providers have seen their situation improve under capitation and do not wish to return to the old payment patterns. In the opinion of Dr. Robert Jamplis of the Palo Alto Clinic Foundation, "We cannot live on fee-for-service alone—it's so low. It costs more to bring up the chart than we are paid to see the patient. I cannot understand the opponents of capitation. [In California,] you just can't live on fee-for-service alone" (Advisory Board Company 1994).

When physicians leave fee-for-service for capitation, they are rewarded for reducing office visits, using fewer diagnostic tests, making fewer referrals to specialists, and cutting back costly hospitalizations. Utilization drops dramatically (see Fig. 3.1).

Unlike the Byzantine arrangements of fee-for-service, claims-based payment, and third-party review, capitation is remarkably straightforward. The essence of capitation is that:

- A single fixed-sum payment is negotiated, covering all care for a defined population.

Figure 3.1. Inpatient Days per 1,000 Population, With and Without Capitation

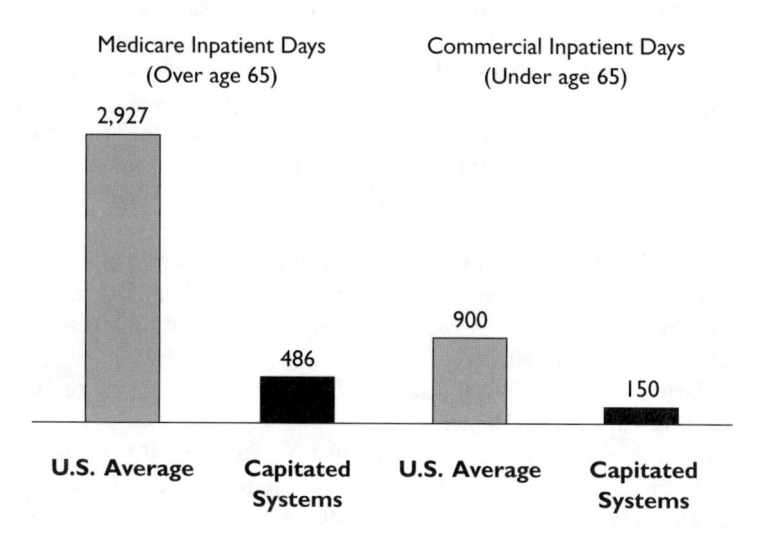

Medicare Inpatient Days (Over age 65)
- U.S. Average: 2,927
- Capitated Systems: 486

Commercial Inpatient Days (Under age 65)
- U.S. Average: 900
- Capitated Systems: 150

Source: "Capitation Strategies," Advisory Board Company, Washington, D.C., 1994, p. 11.

- Each enrollee has a budget—the capitated monthly or annual premium.
- Providers accept the actuarial risk of delivering all needed professional and institutional services.
- Consumers identify a primary physician to manage their care.
- Primary care physicians treat routine health needs and coordinate all referrals to specialists and institutional care.
- Risk pools of funds are set aside for all major categories of professional and institutional care.
- Providers calculate their own internal reimbursement, using subcapitation or fee-for-service.
- Some funds are withheld to insure providers do not overspend.
- Providers police their own utilization and quality.
- Profits or losses are the direct result of provider efficiency.

CAPITATION MAY COVER 15 MILLION ENROLLEES

Capitation is heavily dependent upon the presence of large organized multispecialty medical groups. While it is a predominant West

Coast trend, there are no accurate national statistics on the number of persons enrolled in capitated plans. As of 1994, the Governance Committee, market research division of the Washington, D.C.–based Advisory Board Company, estimated that, at most, 6 percent of the population, or 15 million enrollees, may be covered by fully capitated arrangements (Advisory Board Company 1994).

That estimate assumed almost 40 percent of the nation's 40 million HMO patients may be capitated for all professional services, including staff-model HMO organizations such as the Kaiser Permanente Health Plan. Additional HMO enrollees may be covered by plans that capitate only the primary care physicians. The Governance Committee predicts that 50 percent of all Americans may be fully capitated by the year 2005, at least for all professional services. Market data from InterStudy's national HMO survey indicated that by 1994, 50 percent of HMOs were employing some form of capitation (Hamer 1995).

Capitation is becoming the dominant form of HMO payment to primary care physicians, and the capitation of specialists is accelerating. A national survey of HMOs reported that 45 prepaid plans, some 12.3 percent of all HMOs, predominantly capitate all specialty care (Hamer 1994a). Almost one-third of U.S. prepaid health plans use capitation with at least some physician specialties (see Table 3.1).

UTILIZATION WILL CHANGE OVERNIGHT UNDER CAPITATION

The power of capitation incentives to bring about immediate changes in physician and hospital utilization should not be underestimated. Here is the experience of one integrated system that switched to capitation:

- *In one month,* overall Medicare length of stay dropped from 6.6 to 5.1 days, down 25 percent.
- *In six months,* the length of stay for the top 10 diagnosis-related groups fell from 5 to 4 days, a 25 percent reduction.
- *In one year,* the length of stay for coronary artery bypass grafts fell from 10 days to 6.5, or 35 percent. (Advisory Board Company 1994)

Tracking hospital days at a prestigious California health system showed a managed care–driven downturn of almost 50 percent in eight years for its under-65 commercial HMO patients. Average hospital days per 1,000 enrollees was rolled down from 325 days in 1986 to 220 in 1992, and 185 days in 1994. This utilization

A New Balance of Power for HMOs and Providers

Table 3.1 Forms of Physician Specialty Reimbursement Used by HMOs

Specialty	Fee-for-Service or Discounted Fee-for-Service	Relative Value Scale	Capitation	Salary
Allergy/immunology	65.3%	9.3%	22.4%	3.0%
Anesthesia	74.0	9.9	15.6	0.5
Cardiology	67.1	9.6	21.6	1.6
Dermatology	66.0	9.6	21.1	3.3
Emergency medicine	73.6	9.9	14.9	1.7
Endocrinology	72.1	10.4	15.9	1.6
Gastroenterology	69.4	9.8	18.6	2.2
General surgery	68.0	9.8	19.4	2.7
Hematology/oncology	71.0	9.9	17.5	1.6
Infectious disease	71.2	10.2	16.2	2.5
Nephrology	72.1	10.4	16.1	1.4
Neurology	69.7	10.1	17.8	2.5
Neurosurgery	71.9	10.9	16.1	1.1
Obstetrics/gynecology	67.7	9.6	18.6	4.1
Ophthalmology	66.7	9.3	21.6	2.5
Orthopedics	67.1	10.1	20.0	2.7
Otolaryngology	68.3	9.8	19.9	1.9
Pathology	69.8	8.0	20.9	1.4
Plastic/reconstructive surgery	71.9	10.9	16.4	0.8
Psychiatry	51.5	5.8	39.9	2.8
Pulmonary medicine	70.7	10.1	17.5	1.6
Radiology	68.1	7.4	22.3	2.2
Rheumatology	71.0	10.7	16.4	1.9
Thoracic surgery	71.3	10.1	17.8	0.8
Urology	67.2	9.8	20.8	2.2

Source: Hamer, R. 1994. "HMO Industry Report." InterStudy Competitive Edge. InterStudy Publications, Bloomington, MN.

pattern is not the lowest, either. An aggressive physician group in southern California made even more drastic cuts, reducing under-65 enrollee inpatient days to 155 days in 1993 and 133 in 1994. For a more complete profile, see Table 3.2.

Table 3.2
Utilization Rates per 1,000 Commercial (under-65) HMO Enrollees, With and Without Managed Care

Service	Unmanaged Rate	Moderately Managed Rate	Percentage Decline
Hospital Component			
Inpatient days	430	260	40%
Radiology	375	145	61
Laboratory (output)	500	220	56
Professional Component			
Surgery	1,540	800	48
Radiology	1,250	820	34
Diagnostic testing	480	250	50
Office visits	3,300	2,900	12

Source: Geoffrey Baker, BDC Advisors, San Francisco; cited in "Capitation Strategies," Advisory Board Company, Washington, D.C., 1994, p. 9.

LEARNING THE LANGUAGE OF CAPITATION

Although capitation is new to many healthcare providers, it is not a new concept. Insurance companies have been contracting with employers for almost 60 years on a per capita basis with monthly or annual insurance premiums. What is new is HMOs and insurers sharing a percentage of the capitated premium on a per-enrollee basis with healthcare providers in advance of service.

Much of the language of current capitation arrangements is unfamiliar. Here is a brief overview of key terms.

Capitation. This reimbursement arrangement between payers (HMOs, insurers, employers, governments) and providers (physicians, hospitals) specifies a fixed dollar amount to be paid each month per health plan enrollee, regardless of the services provided.

Per member per month. Capitated payments to providers are typically described in terms of the amount providers will receive per member per month (PMPM) or per year, such as $0.05 to $0.10 PMPM for nephrology.

Risk. With capitation comes risk. Capitation puts providers at risk because they must provide all services defined in the capitation contract, whatever the cost. If providers control their patient care expenditures, they make a profit, and if provider costs rise above the capitated fee, they lose money. Thus providers are rewarded—or penalized—for clinical efficiency.

Gatekeepers. Primary care physicians (those in family practice, internal medicine, pediatrics, and sometimes obstetrics/gynecology) may be paid an additional fee of $1.50 to $4.00 per member per month to act as gatekeepers. Every patient chooses, or is assigned, a primary care physician to coordinate all healthcare needs. Gatekeeper physicians must approve referrals to specialists, as well as expensive diagnostic work and treatments such as surgery or hospitalization.

Risk pools. A percentage of the capitation premium is allocated for each category of service, such as primary care, specialist services, and hospitalization. The fund for each category is the risk pool to be shared by providers, ensuring that not all the money is spent on one category of care, leaving other services underfunded.

Set-asides or *withholds.* To ensure that the capitated dollar will be stretched across the entire year, some percentage of the premium, such as 40 percent, will be set aside or withheld for future allocation. At the end of the quarter, or year, the remaining monies in the withhold pool will be shared with participating providers.

Subcapitation. Some providers may be selected to provide specific services, such as obstetrics, for a per member per month fee. All obstetrics patients are then referred to the designated OB specialists or groups. Subcapitated specialists might receive fees such as these: general surgeons, $0.85 to $1.00 PMPM; orthopedists, $1 to $1.50 PMPM; and obstetrician/gynecologists, $3 to $3.50 PMPM (Mayer 1994).

Carveouts. Carveouts are similiar to subcapitation in that selected services or conditions may be subcontracted to a separate provider network, for a negotiated fee per member per month. Mental health and substance abuse services are often carved out of capitation agreements with other physicians and hospitals.

Bundled or *global fees.* Some high-cost or high-volume services may be subcontracted for a global fee. For example, a global fee for open-heart surgery would cover the surgeon, the anesthesiologist, the hospital, and all related charges.

CAPITATION = LESS MONEY (BUT PROVIDERS CONTROL IT)

Capitation can be very profitable if providers are efficient. But the total of provider payments almost certainly will be less than providers were receiving under fee-for-service and discounted managed care. HMOs and insurers will use the shift to capitation to lower their costs of patient care. John Mayerhofer observes that, in California, "We are converting the current indemnity experience into capitation, and further assuming that since there is overutilization in the current system, any cap that takes 20 percent off the top must, by inference, be a reasonable estimation of what should be spent in the new 'managed care' environment" (Mayerhofer 1994).

Accepting capitation does put providers at economic risk, but two important benefits balance that risk. First, doctors and hospitals retake control of their patients, eliminating outside third-party review from the patient-physician relationship. Second, providers regain control of their economics and the allocation of patient care resources.

HOW CAPITATION WORKS: ANALYSIS OF THE DOLLAR FLOW

For many providers, capitation is a black box. How does it work? Where do the dollars go? Consultants observe there is no set formula, and no two HMOs approach it the same way. Some aspects are still a mystery. Information on subcapitation rates for specialists are considered proprietary information by HMOs and consultants and is not easily discovered. A simple example would be an HMO that has 100 enrollees, each covered by a $100 monthly premium. Yearly premiums total $120,000. Capitation might well allocate dollars, roles, and responsibilities as follows:

Step 1. HMO Administration. The HMO takes $20 off the top for administration, marketing, reinsurance, customer service, and, of course, profit.

Step 2. Physician Capitation. The HMO contracts with a primary care medical group, paying the group $40 per member per month for all medical services. Of that, the medical group retains $10 to cover administrative costs ($7) and ancillary service costs ($3).

Step 3. Primary Care. The enrollee's primary care physician gets the next $10 of the $40. That amount may be somewhat lower if the group chooses to purchase stop-loss insurance from the HMO. Stop-loss protection, which is designed to limit liability beyond a specified amount, would limit the primary care group's risk to perhaps $7,000 per member per year.

Step 4. Specialty Care. The other $20 of the $40 allocated for physician services is placed in a risk pool to cover specialist care. The primary care group pays specialists on a discounted fee-for-service basis, as care occurs. A growing number of primary care groups are now shifting to subcapitation arrangements with single-specialty medical groups or networks.

Step 5. Hospital Capitation. The hospital (or hospital network or multihospital system) gets $40 per member per month for the same number of HMO enrollees that sign up with the physician group. The hospital capitation arrangement typically covers inpatient care, ambulance service, durable medical equipment, and outpatient services provided in the hospital setting.

Step 6. Risk Sharing (and rewards and losses). Assuming 100 capitated lives, the medical group and the hospital each receive $48,000 for the year. The doctors make money if primary care expenses total less than $12,000 and the specialist billings total less than $24,000. Remember that at least some of the $7 for physician group administration can be profit. The hospital has budgeted up to $25,000 per year for inpatient care, $12,000 for outpatient services, and $1,000 for out-of-area hospitalization. Savings in any category result in hospital profit. If the physician group and hospital are joint partners in the capitation scheme, each may share profits or losses with the other, according to a prenegotiated formula. That is why capitation is a risk-sharing arrangement (Mayer 1994).

THE FOOD CHAIN OF CAPITATION PAYMENTS

Managing capitated covered lives fundamentally restructures the dollar-power-responsibility relationships between payers and providers. This new and dynamic relationship may be illustrated through the metaphor of the food chain (see Fig. 3.2).

A new balance of power is emerging between HMOs and providers under capitation. In the food chain, the power of HMOs could weaken substantially, as HMOs turn over utilization management and quality assurance to primary care physicians or integrated physician-hospital organizations. HMOs are acknowledging their limits in cost containment by switching to capitation as their chief strategy for controlling costs.

But there are major benefits to HMOs when they put providers under capitation. With capitation, the HMO can shift risk almost completely to the providers. High-dollar rewards will go to the *integrator of care*, whichever entity controls costs and referrals in the food chain. In the past, that power was held by the insurance company or HMO. In the future, organized physicians or integrated health systems/PHOs will capture the integrator role.

Five Stages of Managed Care

Figure 3.2. The New Food Chain of Payer-Provider Relations under Capitation

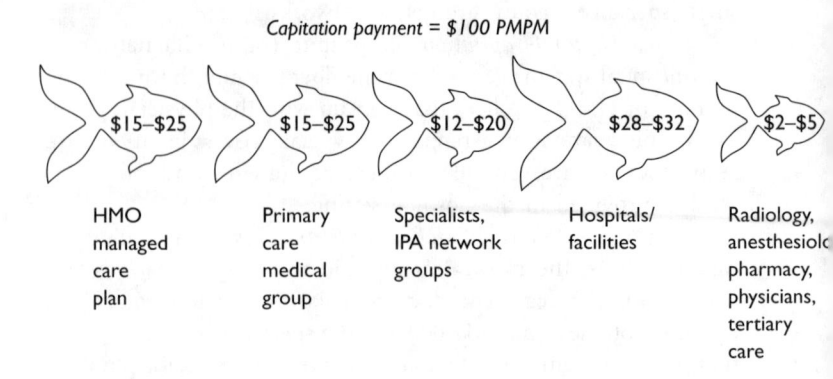

Capitation payment = $100 PMPM

| $15–$25 | $15–$25 | $12–$20 | $28–$32 | $2–$5 |

| HMO managed care plan | Primary care medical group | Specialists, IPA network groups | Hospitals/ facilities | Radiology, anesthesiolc pharmacy, physicians, tertiary care |

Source: Health Forecasting Group, April 1994.

The food chain of capitation is likely to favor physicians over hospitals. As HMOs and insurers expand their use of capitation, they are shifting cash flow from institutional providers to physician providers. Further, HMO capitation patterns favor primary care physicians over specialists. Strong primary care groups like southern California's Friendly Hills Medical Group or the Huntington Provider Group can get 85 to 89 percent of the global capitation premium covering all health services, cutting the HMO share down to 11 to 15 percent. One result has been an explosion of nearly two dozen for-profit physician management corporations that purchase primary care physicians and groups, hoping to capture the role of integrator of care in the capitation food chain.

HOSPITALS ORGANIZE FOR CAPITATION

Hospitals and physicians are now organizing statewide and regional managed care networks in anticipation of a market dominated by capitation. The key factor in provider conversion to capitation is the joint acceptance of risk by a physician-hospital organization. Signing a contract for capitated lives is a watershed moment in relations between hospitals and their medical staffs. It commits doctors and the administration and board to a new partnership of mutual trust and shared responsibility. Only with capitation does the independent medical staff become economically aligned with the hospital. Managing utilization, costs, and clinical outcomes will be the critical success factors.

Hospitals and physicians are now aggressively preparing for capitation. In a national survey for *Modern Healthcare* by Quorum Health Resources of Nashville, Tennessee, some 54 percent of surveyed hospitals were developing PHOs (see Fig. 3.3). Study director Allen Fine, currently the senior manager, Healthcare Consulting Practice, Ernst & Young, in Chicago, observes: "We're beginning to see hospitals and their medical staffs move beyond the rhetoric to develop collaborative organizations with common goals" (Kenkel 1994).

About 16 percent of the 400 surveyed hospitals had replaced an existing independent practice association with a more integrated form of physician-hospital organization. On average, hospitals put up 75 percent of the initial capital. Physicians are at risk for their contributed investments. Many of the new PHOs share governance fifty-fifty with physicians.

For example, the Charleston (West Virginia) Area Medical Center created a PHO with an eight-member board made up of four physicians and four hospital members. At least one of the physicians must be from primary care. Some 350 physicians, about 75 percent of the hospital's medical staff, have signed up with CareLink. The goal of the PHO was to tap into the emerging managed care marketplace in West Virginia. Doctors hope the PHO will help them improve their patient mix and cash flow. CareLink doubled in enrollment in the first two years, from 11,000 in 1992 to over 23,000 in 1993. As a result of its positive experience with capitation, the Charleston hospital is now seeking an HMO license and planning to target midsized and small employer groups with fewer than 100 employees. Plans call for the PHO to be

Figure 3.3. Physicians and Hospitals Organize for Capitation

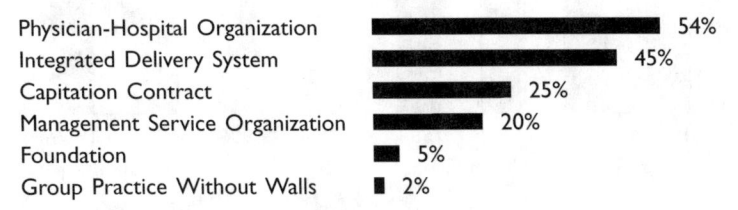

Physician-Hospital Organization	54%
Integrated Delivery System	45%
Capitation Contract	25%
Management Service Organization	20%
Foundation	5%
Group Practice Without Walls	2%

Source: Created from data presented in Kenkel, P. J. 1994. "The Systematic Approach: Physician-Hospital Collaborations Increase, Work to Capture Managed-Care Contracts." Modern Healthcare 24 (14): 59–65.

Five Stages of Managed Care

absorbed by the HMO, with the hospital providing capital for the transition.

PHYSICIAN GROUPS WILL EMBRACE CAPITATION

American medicine is about to be restructured by two tremendous shifts, both moving in the same direction: (1) group practice and (2) capitation. Medical groups are expanding rapidly to play a lead role in managed care. The number of primary care physicians in large, urban group practices is on the rise (see Fig. 3.4), and so is the percent of their capitated business, according to a national survey for *Hospitals & Health Networks* by Atlanta-based consultants Hamilton/KSA, in cooperation with the American Group Practice Association (Montague 1994).

Larger medical groups positioning for capitation are not just a California trend. In Temple, Texas, the Scott and White Clinic is a 405-physician group practice with 11 satellite clinics, a hospital, and an HMO. About 35 percent of the group's business is capitated, and a third of its physicians are primary care practitioners (Montague 1994). Scott and White is accelerating its recruitment of primary care physicians to assist in managed care and capitation.

Figure 3.4. Group Practices Grow, Take on Capitation

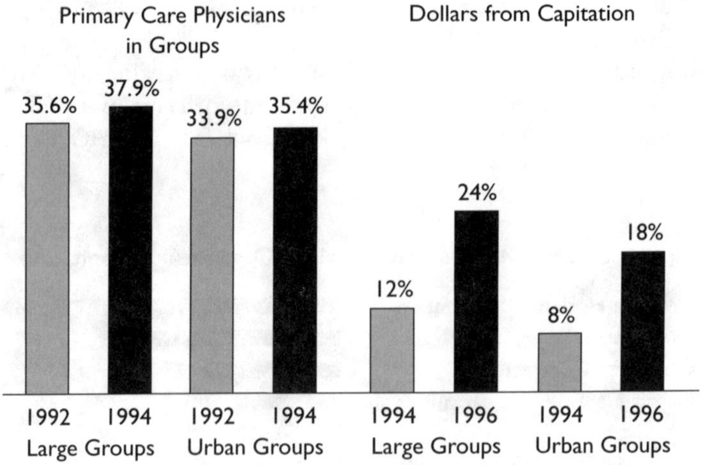

Primary Care Physicians in Groups:
- 1992 Large Groups: 35.6%
- 1994 Large Groups: 37.9%
- 1992 Urban Groups: 33.9%
- 1994 Urban Groups: 35.4%

Dollars from Capitation:
- 1994 Large Groups: 12%
- 1996 Large Groups: 24%
- 1994 Urban Groups: 8%
- 1996 Urban Groups: 18%

Source: Adapted from data by Hamilton/KSA; cited in Montague, J. 1994. "Precision Maneuvers." Hospitals & Health Networks 68 (1): 26–33.

The same pattern is evolving in Everett, Washington, a Seattle suburb. The Everett Clinic, a 115-physician group, has increased its primary care staff from 30 percent to 40 percent in response to managed care.

The shift to capitation is strongest in the West, where more than half of physician groups report that managed care and capitation constitute the largest percent of their business. On a national basis, 75 percent of physician groups report that fee-for-service is still their primary business, but all regions expect that managed care will constitute at least 50 percent of their revenues within two years.

HOW DOCTORS CAN TELL IF AN HMO CAPITATION CONTRACT WILL BE PROFITABLE

Many U.S. physicians are still skeptical about managed care. They are fearful of losing income and patient control, and have no idea whether a particular HMO agreement may be profitable. "A lot of doctors are signing up with HMOs to be competitive, but they have no idea whether they will make or lose money on those patients," reports David Scroggins, a practice management consultant in Cincinnati (Walker 1992).

Calculating the potential for profits or losses with managed care begins with a strong working knowledge of physician practice costs. With a capitation agreement, the physician practice should know its per member per month costs for treating similar patients. The biggest problem is that physician practices often have no data. In capitation contracting with a typical commercial HMO (i.e., one whose patients are under age 65), key data elements, exclusive of Medicare and Medicaid patients, include:

- total number of active fee-for-service patients;
- number of annual fee-for-service visits;
- type of services;
- net revenues per service (billed charges minus discounts and uncollectibles); and
- average overhead operating cost per patient visit.

Every physician practice should profile the age and sex of its patients. Many HMO enrolled groups contain an above-average number of families with young children. HMO copayments are often low, so the number of primary care visits such patients may demand is often higher than a typical family physician might experience. More and more HMOs are offering age-adjusted and sex-adjusted capitation rates. The more a physician practice patient base resembles the HMO enrollees, the closer the doctors' experience will be to the HMO patients' potential demand.

Coverage of tests and ancillary costs is often overlooked. Doctors should know exactly what tests and other ancillary services the contract requires the capitated physician to cover. For example, a pediatric group was hit with higher-than-expected immunization costs when a product liability suit drove up the cost of vaccines. The next year, the group asked that immunization be covered at actual cost. The HMO compensated by cutting the capitation rate, but after the second year, the pediatricians did very well (Walker 1992).

Management of specialist referrals is a high-cost item. In the past, HMOs often placed primary care physicians in a dilemma by withholding funds from primary care doctors for specialist risk pools. But doctors resented when withhold funds were not returned at year-end. Now HMOs are shifting instead to bonus arrangements, to reward a primary care physician or group when specialist referrals are under a specified number. This may reduce the capitation payment, but at least under the bonus plan, primary care physicians are guaranteed to get the full reimbursement instead of suffering any withhold. A stop-loss provision can reduce a physician's or groups' liability, but will be an offset to the capitation rate. Usually, the more patients in the contract, the greater risk the doctors can afford, advises Edward Grab, consultant with The Health Care Group in Plymouth Meeting, Pennsylvania (Walker 1992). If a group has 500 versus 50 HMO capitated enrollees, one high-cost patient is not such a risk factor.

There is more to a capitation contract than just the profit-loss analysis. Primary care physicians should examine other doctors on the HMO's local panel. If most primary care physicians on the panel are family practitioners, then internists may get more of the complicated cases. Doctors should also review what specialists are included in the specialty referral panel to determine if the practice will be comfortable referring to them.

MEDICAID CAPITATION CONTRACTING: NEW MECHANISM FOR HEALTH REFORM

A nationwide wave of Medicaid capitation contracting may act as the training wheels for national health reform. According to HCFA, risk-based Medicaid contracting programs have been growing at an annual rate of 12 percent for the last five years (Kenkel 1994). HCFA's Office of Managed Care reports that more than 5 million Medicaid recipients are now enrolled in 200 capitated plans, some

15 percent of the 32.9 million Medicaid beneficiaries on a national basis. InterStudy reports that Medicaid HMOs are growing fast, by 23.1 percent in 1995 (Hamer 1996). The growth took place in all regions, with federally qualified HMOs picking up 61.2 percent of the new Medicaid HMO enrollees. Large, national HMOs were more likely than independent HMOs or Blue Cross/Blue Shield to market aggressively to Medicaid beneficiaries.

Medicaid capitation experiments give providers some experience with government-sponsored capitation programs. In this post-reform scenario, states will merge their Medicaid and uninsured populations for risk-based contracting. Providers and insurers bid to become qualified health reform/Medicaid contractors, as choices for Medicaid enrollees. In addition to Washington, the states of Michigan, Tennessee, Kentucky, and Delaware have enacted or initiated Medicaid contracting programs. More than a dozen states have sought or received HCFA waivers to shift their Medicaid population to capitation.

At the local level, Medicaid capitation is working. In Seattle, the Highline Community Hospital developed a physician-hospital organization to participate in Washington state's new capitated Medicaid program. With their insurance partner, Healthy Options, Highline is grossing $10.6 million annually, based on capitated payments of $130 per enrollee for 7,000 covered lives. Highline's 100 participating physicians are helping control hospital and emergency costs in a shared-risk arrangement. In its first three months with the state contract, Highline saved an estimated $350,000, largely due to a reduction in emergency room use. Highline has divided the 25 primary care physicians into five panels for comparison purposes to analyze patterns of referral for specialty care. Doctors are monitoring and managing their performance in the new arrangement, and Highline's PHO is prospering under Medicaid capitation.

MEDICARE HMO WINDOW OF OPPORTUNITY FOR PROVIDER CAPITATION

The nation's 33 million senior citizens are the high-priority targets of Medicare HMOs. The Medicare HMO window of opportunity is opening now for providers to become engaged in at-risk capitation contracting. Capitating Medicare beneficiaries could change the fortunes of hundreds of U.S. hospitals that are heavily dependent upon Medicare fee-for-service patients today. Hospitals and physicians unwilling to jump into capitation could lose their

Medicare patients to other providers who are willing and able to manage risk with Medicare HMOs.

Medicare risk contracting had a rocky beginning. Authorized in 1985, only 1 million Medicare beneficiaries were signed up by the end of 1986. Three years later, Medicare HMO enrollment had reached a modest level of 1.5 million. Some Medicare risk plans were successful, but others struggled and failed. Successful plans were generally larger and had more sophisticated utilization management systems and competitive pricing. Less successful Medicare HMOs had hospital use rates as high as 3,500 patients per 1,000 enrollees, compared with rates of 1,000 to 1,250 patients per 1,000 for profitable plans.

Medicare HMOs are now gaining real momentum, with growth rates of 23.1 percent in 1995, according to InterStudy (Hamer 1996). The number of commercial HMOs participating in Medicare capitation is growing. Almost one-third of all HMOs now offer Medicare products. Growth is still concentrated in California, Florida, Oregon, Texas, Minnesota, and New York. InterStudy characterizes Medicare capitation as "one of the four fastest-growing product areas" for HMOs (Hamer 1996, 39).

Analysis of performance among Medicare HMOs identified capitation of the primary care physician as the critical strategy in at-risk contracting for Medicare enrollees. The most successful primary physicians have been involved in Medicare capitation for at least one year. Many of these doctors had been pioneers of managed care in their communities. Primary care physicians share capitation for primary care, as well as a portion of the specialist and hospital care pools. Capitation does make a difference in the management of Medicare patients. Physician office staff who would have been billing under fee-for-service arrangements instead are reassigned to assist the primary physicians in case management and care coordination.

The cash flow from Medicare HMO patients to capitated providers can be substantial. In Seattle, Washington, a Medicare HMO enrollee in King County produced a capitation payment of $363.49 per member per month (Kenkel 1994). California-based PacifiCare, one of the nation's most successful Medicare HMOs, is contracting at risk in Washington and a half-dozen other states. PacifiCare's Medicare HMO, the Secure Horizons plan, has enrolled 318,000 Medicare beneficiaries.

Medicare HMOs will emerge as major players in rural areas, where many seniors are located. In Lawton, Oklahoma, an innovative Medicare risk plan is being launched by a rural health network of eight hospitals organized by the Commanche Regional Medical Center. This is an experiment to demonstrate the feasibility of the capitation model in a rural network. The rural network is now taking capitation, beginning with primary care providers, and Medicare at-risk contracting has been launched. The entire provider network should soon be under capitation.

A CAPITATION MODEL FOR MENTAL HEALTH SERVICES

Capitation models for managing mental health services are highly promising. In arrangements known as "carveouts," mental health providers and specialized managed care plans are subcontracting to manage mental health care. Even patients with serious mental health disorders can be managed in capitated programs.

In California, two pilot projects with community-based mental health providers are successful demonstrations of managed costs and improved outcomes (Hargreaves 1992). The California legislature initiated a program creating integrated services agencies to manage the care of patients rated as disabled due to mental disorders. Experiments in rural Stanislaus County and in Long Beach, an urban setting, showed that the integrated services agencies could manage these more difficult mentally ill patients in community settings under capitation rates of $13,500 to $15,000 per year, well below the cost of hospitalization in state facilities or fee-for-service programs.

LOOKING FORWARD: HEALTH PROMOTION FOR CAPITATION SUCCESS

Critics of capitation worry that providers will be tempted to skimp on care, defer referrals for more costly specialty care, or even systematically deny access to patients, via limited hours of service, long waits, and months-long delays for specialist appointments. Meyerhofer (1994) predicts that, "As capitation decreases and cash flows are squeezed, delivery systems are going to be forced to ration. Whether it is through overt rationing or covert rationing, we are going to have rationing."

Health promotion, however, is the ultimate strategy for long-term success under capitation. Here is the financing mechanism and incentives that the wellness movement has lacked. Under fee-for-service, providers never got paid for promoting health—only for curing disease. That is changing. The upside potential for capitation is that providers will work to optimize a patient's health, because prevention is the ultimate demand-reduction strategy. Healthy patients need fewer services and are at lower risk for high-cost acute-care incidents such as heart attacks and strokes.

Capitated providers will identify patients who carry health risks such as hypertension or diabetes, as well as enrollees with poor health habits, such as smoking. High-risk patients can be successfully placed in case management programs and provided with education and support to modify their health risks.

For example, providers can succeed in Medicare at-risk contracts if they successfully identify and manage high-risk seniors. Gerontologist Peter Yedidia of San Francisco–based Geriatric Health Systems estimates that 15 percent of Medicare patients need case management and continuous monitoring (Yedidia 1994). "High-risk" means patients with several health conditions that interact to create more potential need for healthcare. This potential risk can be identified in a mailed, self-administered patient questionnaire that has 90 percent response rate, according to Yedidia. As expected, some 38.7 percent of the "oldest old," those over age 85, have the greatest likelihood for high risk. But most Medicare enrollees are under age 75, so Yedidia cautions at-risk providers to identify the most unhealthy patients at all age levels.

STRATEGIES FOR PROVIDERS, HMOs, AND SUPPLIERS

Providers

Providers should start organizing now for capitation. Hospitals and physicians cannot wait until capitation arrives in their market before developing structures such as PHOs, management service organizations (MSOs), and managed care divisions. Everything starts with the doctors. Committed physicians willing to manage their own costs and quality are the key to successful capitation management. Community health information networks (CHINs) that link all providers with clinical and financial data are a wise investment. At this early stage, buyers will be smarter than sellers. HMOs and insurers will have more information on capitation pricing than providers. Buyers already have set prices per member per month for every service, physician specialty, and procedure. This has all been worked out. Providers who fail to secure expert consultation are likely to face capitation deals that do not cover provider costs.

HMOs

Already, HMOs are discovering the benefits of capitation—absolute control and predictability of costs. HMOs should be able to reduce their costs of care by 10 to 15 percent and more. The hidden benefit of capitation is that HMOs may now substantially reduce their overhead costs to 5 to 6 percent of the premium. Under capitation, HMOs can dismantle their expensive infrastructure. Gone is much of the detail work of utilization management, quality assurance, provider credentialing, and network management. HMO overhead costs could be cut by 25 to 40 percent or more. Under capitation, the providers perform all these functions. To ensure quality and customer service, however, HMOs must require providers to compile data such as the HEDIS indicators and to submit reports according to HMO specifications.

Suppliers

Capitation is a new world for suppliers. Producers of supplies, materials, and equipment may be in for a shock. All the incentives under capitation will drive use of their products down by 15 to 50 percent, in some categories, over the next five to seven years. This is the time for customer partnerships. Providers and their group purchasing organizations will need help from suppliers in fine-tuning every aspect of provider costs. As providers develop standardized protocols for each procedure and diagnosis, suppliers can assist in standardizing the supply and equipment components. For example, the standardization of orthopedic hip implant devices can save $300,000 to $500,000 for an active orthopedic service. Suppliers can react with price cuts to protect customer loyalty, but that is only a short-term solution and does not solve the problem of declining demand. In the future, some suppliers will participate in capitation or premium-sharing arrangements. More meaningfully, suppliers, manufacturers, and distributors must be "part of the solution" in the conversion to capitation.

SOURCES

Advisory Board Company. 1994. *Capitation Strategies*. Washington, D.C.: The Governance Committee.

Hamer, R. 1994. "HMO Industry Report." *InterStudy Competitive Edge* 4 (1): 1–136.

———. 1995. "HMO Industry Report, Part II." *InterStudy Competitive Edge* 5 (1): 1–126.

———. 1996. "HMO Industry Report, Part II." *InterStudy Competitive Edge* 6 (1): 1–136.

Hargreaves, W. A. 1992. "A Capitation Model for Providing Mental Health Services in California." *Hospital and Community Psychiatry* 43 (3): 275–77.

Kenkel, P. S. 1994. "Physician-Hospital Collaborations Increase, Work to Capture Managed Care Contracts." *Modern Healthcare* 24 (14): 59–65.

Mayer, D. 1994. "Coping with Capitation." *Northern California Medicine* 5 (2): 19, 24–25.

Mayerhofer, J. 1994. "Capitation Will Lead to Rationing." *Northern California Medicine* 5 (2): 25.

Montague, J. 1994. "Precision Maneuvers." *Hospitals & Health Networks* 68 (1): 26–33.

Walker, L. 1992. "How to Tell If An HMO Will Make You Money." *Medical Economics* 69 (22): 161–68.

Yedidia, P. 1994. "Providers Can Succeed with Medicare Risk Contracts." *Northern California Medicine* 5 (2): 22–23.

CHAPTER 4

Physician-Hospital Strategies for Capitation

Back East, the HMOs are trying to put off capitation for a while. In California, I think the Genie's already out of the bottle.

Chief Executive Officer, Large Multispecialty Group
(Advisory Board Company 1994)

NO ONE in healthcare should get comfortable because health reform failed in Washington, D.C. Market-driven reform is jolting the health field. Just as healthcare providers and suppliers are adjusting to managed care, the market is entering a new world of capitation, risk assumption, gatekeepers, employer direct contracting, physician-hospital organizations, integrated delivery networks, report cards, and disease management.

Healthcare in the United States is a deal-a-week environment, with new partners and business ventures. Insurance companies and HMOs are purchasing physician practices. Blue Cross plans are buying hospitals or merging with them. Hospitals and doctors are starting HMOs. Everyone is repositioning for capitation.

In this managed care market, health reform is only an accelerator. The trigger factor is the rapid conversion of commercial health insureds and Medicare beneficiaries to HMO enrollees. If health reform is ever implemented, perhaps after the year 2000, the new health plan for the nation's 30 to 40 million uninsured will probably be an HMO. HMOs will also scramble to enroll Medicare eligibles, offering them low copayments and cheap prescription drugs. The nation's employers are converting their health plans to HMOs, which offer an estimated 15 to 25 percent price advantage over preferred provider organizations and managed indemnity plans (Coile 1994). Two out of three Americans who are insured through their workplace are enrolled in managed care plans (Eckholm 1994).

A new breed of HMOs is emerging—for-profit, very aggressive, and willing to compete on price. For-profit HMOs now serve more than 55 percent of all HMO enrollees in "pure" and open-ended plans combined, according to InterStudy (Hamer 1995). Companies like U.S. Healthcare in Pennsylvania, United Healthcare in Minneapolis, and PacifiCare in southern California are expanding rapidly through mergers, acquisitions, and enrollment growth. The strategies for managing risk that emerged in southern California and other managed care hot-spots will radically transform U.S. hospitals and physicians over the next several years.

PHYSICIANS LEAD THE CONVERSION TO CAPITATION

Doctors are leading the conversion to managed care. In Los Angeles, seven large physician organizations controlled 75 pecent of the HMO patients (Eckholm 1994). The rapid conversion from production-related payment to at-risk capitation is driven by physician group practices that are enthusiastically embracing capitated arrangements. In California, some 15 medical groups obtained 90 to 95 percent of their revenues from capitation (Advisory Board Company 1994).

Managed care plans are negotiating discounts on procedures like open-heart surgery. In California, "the incomes of specialists are dropping like stones," according to David Langness of the Hospital Council of Southern California (Eckholm 1994). Some 75 percent of Californians and 25 percent of Medicare seniors are enrolled in managed care plans. In Massachusetts, Minnesota, and parts of the West, more than a third of the population is enrolled in HMOs.

Once physicians are capitated and assume risk, the results are drastic cuts in hospital admissions and lengths of inpatient stay. One integrated system slashed Medicare inpatient care by 1.5 days in the first month after capitating the physicians. Inpatient days per 1,000 population could drop more than 300 percent (see Fig. 4.1). California is setting the pace. West Coast integrated systems and physician groups operate with only 140 to 220 inpatient days per

Figure 4.1 U.S. Hospital Inpatient Days per 1,000 Population under Managed Care

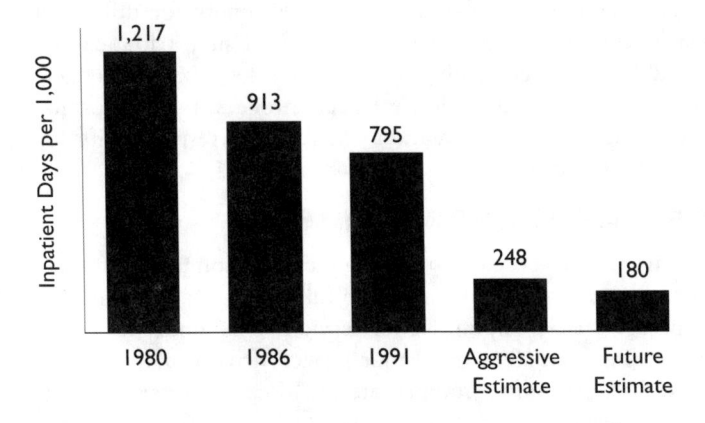

[Bar chart showing Inpatient Days per 1,000:
- 1980: 1,217
- 1986: 913
- 1991: 795
- Aggressive Estimate: 248
- Future Estimate: 180]

Source: "Capitation Strategies," Advisory Board Company, Washington, D.C., 1994, p. 29.

1,000 commercial enrollees, compared with 280 to 325 days for integrated systems on the East Coast and in the Midwest. The national average is almost 500 days!

Aggressive managed care plans and capitated medical groups are continuing to push hospital utilization rates to new lows, as doctors learn that assuming risk means managing utilization:

- Nationally, hospital use rate for commercial (under age 65) HMO enrollees has been cut from 486 days per 1,000 to 150 days.
- Medicare (over age 65) enrollees average over 2,900 hospital days per 1,000, while West Coast physician groups are managing their Medicare HMO covered lives with 700 to 800 days per 1,000.
- Emergency room utilization has been slashed from 357 visits per 1,000 on a national average to 145 to 165 per 1,000 in integrated healthcare systems.
- Group Health of Puget Sound, a Seattle-based HMO, lowered prescription drug costs from $102 to $73 per member.
- The Fallon Community Health Plan in Massachusetts lowered the rates for cesarean-section deliveries from the state average of 24 percent to 15 percent. (Advisory Board Company 1994)

The secret to cost-effective management of risk under capitation is physician leadership in the PHOs. One large healthcare system cut Medicare length of stay by 1.5 days in a matter of months after the system transferred responsibility for utilization management to its affiliated medical clinic. Using a foundation, the healthcare system had built a covered-lives base of 60,000 commercial and 7,000 Medicare HMO enrollees, put its hospital and physicians on full capitation, then shifted responsibility for utilization control of the hospital to the doctors.

CAPITATING SPECIALISTS

The conventional approach to making the transition to capitation is to put the primary care physicians on full capitation, but continue to pay the specialists on fee-for-service. This does not work well. Leaving specialists on fee-for-service drives up utilization, as specialists attempt to compensate for discounted payments by increasing services. A study of 2,000 HMO patients showed that capitated primary care physicians successfully reduced admissions from 154 to 139 per 1,000 enrollees, but hospital charges rose $250 per discharge and length of inpatient stay climbed from 4.0 to 4.6 days, as specialists took advantage of fee-for-service incentives (Stearns et al. 1992).

The new economics of specialty physician payment will be fixed payments per member per month paid in advance of treatment. Capitation payments vary by specialty, by region, and by group, depending upon the negotiated scope of service (see Fig. 4.2). The capitation agreement with specialists specifically identifies those services and tests to be covered.

Specialty capitation rates may vary 50 to 100 percent, according to the range of services covered and the historical utilization rates of the enrolled population. For example, the cardiology rate, which may or may not include invasive procedures, may vary from $0.31 to $1.12 per member per month. Similarly, orthopedics may vary from $1.00 to $1.50.

Giving specialists the incentives inherent in capitation can have far-reaching results. The Advisory Board Company (1994) describes a 12-member cardiology group that began to take capitation. The group restructured its practice by selecting four cardiologists with a bias toward noninvasive treatments to act as gatekeepers. All referrals from primary care practitioners are now routed through these four cardiologists. The cardiology gatekeepers do all the work ups. Inappropriate patients are referred back to the PCPs, while appropriately referred patients are assigned to the cardiology group's various subspecialists.

Figure 4.2 Capitation Payments by Specialty (Average per Member per Month for commercial HMO patients)

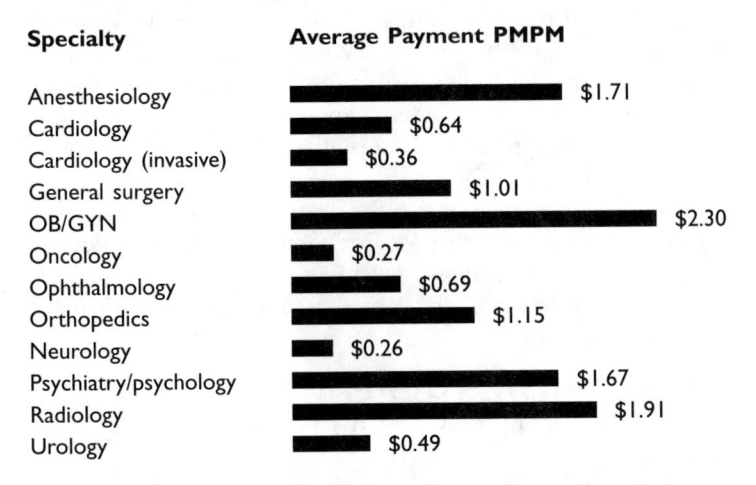

Specialty	Average Payment PMPM
Anesthesiology	$1.71
Cardiology	$0.64
Cardiology (invasive)	$0.36
General surgery	$1.01
OB/GYN	$2.30
Oncology	$0.27
Ophthalmology	$0.69
Orthopedics	$1.15
Neurology	$0.26
Psychiatry/psychology	$1.67
Radiology	$1.91
Urology	$0.49

Source: The HMO Executive Salary Survey, Warren Surveys, Rockford, IL, 1993; cited in "Capitation Strategies," Advisory Board Company, Washington, D.C., 1994, p. 94.

Cardiologists now spend more time with their primary care referral sources. Because of regular telephone consultations, cardiology referrals from PCPs are markedly down, and so are costs per case. Shorter consultations are needed, once patients have been worked up by the cardiology gatekeepers, and fewer tests are used. For example, stress testing of hypertensive patients has been slashed 95 percent, by reducing the test interval from four times each year to once every five years for patients whose other cardiology indicators are within expected ranges (Advisory Board Company 1994).

ERA OF CAPITATION ARRIVED OVERNIGHT IN ATLANTA

Capitation arrived in the heart of the Old South. The Wyeth Insurance Company has created an exclusive surgery network for metropolitan Atlanta, covering general, vascular, and colon and rectal surgery (Advisory Board Company 1994). Doctors were invited to compete for at-risk insurance agreements.

Under this scheme, physicians were paid by capitation, and providers bid for the business. Only 40 of the original HMO panel of 150 surgeons were chosen, almost a 75 percent reduction. To assist Atlanta-area providers to compete, Wyeth held a bidders' conference for physicians and hospitals, but deadlines were short. The insurer gave providers barely two weeks to respond. Surgeons quickly formed networks with multiple locations around Atlanta and established quality management and utilization management programs. As billing would be via electronic claims submission, doctors were expected to have computerized management information systems, appointment scheduling, and medical records.

Atlanta braced for more capitation strategies. Two other health insurers announced plans to capitate physician specialists, including surgeons, cardiologists, orthopedists, obstetricians, gynecologists, neurologists, and oncologists. Doctors scrambled to develop economic relationships in clinical networks, and the time frame once again is very short.

CALIFORNIA HOSPITAL THRIVES ON CAPITATION

Hospitals fear they will be losers—not winners—under capitation. This is not necessarily the case. Downey Community Hospital, in southern California, radically restructured for a capitated marketplace. Aggressive cost reduction was balanced with a proactive marketing approach with its physicians. The payoff for this 350-bed hospital was thousands of covered lives, lower inpatient days, and millions in new revenues. Downey CEO Carl Westerhoff changed his organization's paradigm. "We don't view ourselves as being in the hospital business, we view ourselves as being in the health care delivery business." In a market with over 200 hospitals, Westerhoff says bluntly, "Nobody needs you" (Advisory Board Company 1994).

So what do hospitals have to offer? The first asset is capital. In a changing marketplace, hospitals have a strong capital base to finance new directions. The second asset is a critical mass of management. Downey Community Hospital proactively marketed the hospital and its physicians to HMOs, capitated physician groups, and other managed care buyers. Here is how they did it:

- A cost-savings committee studied all departments for savings potential.
- Capital investments in facilities improvements were completed before the change in Medicare pass-through reimbursement.
- All units used flexible staffing, tied to occupancy.
- Management reductions and the substitution of midlevel nursing staff for RNs lowered nursing costs.
- Streamlined paperwork consolidated 15 patient care forms into a single record.

- The pharmacy tightened the hospital's formulary through cost-benefit analysis of drugs.
- All supplies and equipment were ordered through group purchasing agreements.
- All scheduled patients received same-day admissions.
- All patients were put under centralized case management.
- A physician was assigned as team leader for care management of each patient's entire stay.
- Weekly utilization meetings coordinated the efforts of physicians, home health providers, discharge planners, utilization reviewers, and business office personnel. (Cochrane 1993)

The hospital's strategies for assuming and managing risk with its physicians yielded dramatic, positive bottom-line results. Medicare HMO inpatient utilization dropped from 1,700 bed days per 1,000 enrollees in 1990 to 1,100 in 1993, while commercial HMO inpatient utilization fell from 250 inpatient days to 180. Managed care revenues soared. Annual revenues climbed from $53 million in 1990 to $97 million in 1993, and net revenues improved 400 percent, from $2 million to $8 million. Downey Community Hospital's experience in assuming and managing risk demonstrates the possibility of success in capitated markets.

EIGHT STRATEGIES FOR CAPITATION

The Advisory Board Company (1994) outlines and ranks eight strategies for capitation contracting (see Table 4.1). This summary of capitation strategies is made available by special permission of the Advisory Board Company.

Strategy 1. Spot-Market Contracting

"Spot marketing" is a term from the commodities market that means selling at the last minute, usually for a low price. A hospital agrees to accept a discounted per diem payment rate from an HMO or capitated physician group that subcontracts for hospital services. In effect, the hospital bed day becomes a commodity. The hospital has no control over future volume in such arrangements, and the buyer is under no obligation to use the hospital.

Is spot-market contracting a viable strategy? Probably not. Hospital chief financial officers may claim that, by spot-market contracting, they are aggressively pricing the hospital's marginal capacity, to fill remaining beds with any patients, even if payment rates are low. But this ignores the reality that this type of contracting

Table 4.1
Ranking Eight Capitation Contracting Models

Models	Advisory Board Company Rating
Facilities Contracting	
Spot-market contracting	C−
Hospital subcapitation	C
Specialty Capitation	
Carveout capitation	B
Chronic care capitation	B−
Medicare risk contracting	A
Full-Risk Capitation	
Partnership capitation	A
Network capitation	A
System capitation	A

Source: "Capitation Strategies," Advisory Board Company, Washington, D.C., 1994, p. 4.

is not a sustainable strategy. With a surplus of hospital beds in most states, this is a buyer's market. Further, as physicians are increasingly shifted to capitation, their incentives will continue to reduce hospital utilization, leaving hospitals helpless in the face of HMOs and capitated medical groups who will demand deeper discounts.

Spot-market contracting and hospital subcapitation (Strategy 2) are short-term strategies intended to fill beds. While they may provide some transitional revenues, they are shortsighted and do not position hospitals in favorable niches or take over the function of integrator of care. The winners in markets shifting to capitation will be those hospitals that see the window of opportunity to create a multilevel delivery system with an integrated physician delivery network that can assume and manage risk in capitation agreements.

Strategy 2. Hospital Subcapitation

Under "subcapitation," hospitals move into capitation arrangements, but as subcontractors and vendors. Hospitals subcontract to provide services in their facilities on a capitated basis, but someone else—usually an integrated system or physician group—actually holds and manages the capitation contract. The positive aspect of this arrangement is that it puts hospitals on the inside of capitated agreements, with predictable revenues, and in a position to gain from their own internal efficiencies and cost management efforts. But the negative reality is that another provider organization holds the real contract, and the freestanding hospital is quite vulnerable in the relationship.

Once physicians are capitated, they have an enormous interest in reducing institutional care. The Governance Committee predicted that a 400-bed hospital could see a $17 million decline in marginal profits (Advisory Board Company 1994). The revenue losses deepen as HMO penetration rises:

- 30 percent HMO penetration = $7.2–$9.9 million reduction.
- 40 percent HMO penetration = $9.7–$13.3 million reduction.
- 50 percent HMO penetration = $12.1–$16.7 million reduction.

There are ways to sweeten the subcapitation deal for hospitals as utilization drops. An added incentive in some hospital subcapitation agreements is a provision to share in savings from reduced utilization through a risk pool or facilities budget. For example, an inpatient fund established by the HMO or capitated medical group may be charged on a per diem basis as hospital services are rendered, with any surplus being shared fifty-fifty between the HMO and the hospital or physician organization.

Given a choice between per diem payments and subcapitation, the choice of capitation is a "no-brainer." Hospitals must convert as many per diem HMO and insurance contracts to subcapitation as rapidly as possible. Hospital costs are going to be cut, and hospitals should get in on any gain-sharing from the risk pool so that they will benefit from the savings generated by lowering utilization.

Strategy 3. Carveout Capitation

Carveout contracting involves centers of excellence. The hospital contracts to provide specialized hospital services in defined clinical niches. This capitation strategy pays hospitals on a per member per month basis to provide a well-defined range of specialty services that are carved out of a comprehensive hospital services agreement. This has been a popular strategy for subcontracting mental health care ($4.50 PMPM), substance abuse treatment ($1.16), pharmacy ($8.70) and home health services ($0.09). Occupational health and dental and vision care are other popular carveouts.

HMOs and insurance companies often carve out cardiology services, especially invasive cardiology, transplants, ophthalmology, and expensive tests such as MRIs. The four most popular targets for niche carveouts—cardiology, oncology, orthopedics, and ophthalmology—account for some 33 percent of the typical hospital's inpatient days.

Hospitals need to mobilize their best assets—specialized medical services—and the window of opportunity may be small. Specialty carveouts may not be contracted out twice. In transitional Stage 2 and Stage 3 managed care markets, payers are either capitating hospitals for specialty care already or are negotiating capitation rates with specialists. Although the carveout strategy alone will not sustain an academic medical center or regional hospital, it is a significant business opportunity for those hospitals with recognized specialty expertise.

Strategy 4. Chronic Care Capitation

Chronic care niches may be deeper and broader than the carveout market for such specialized procedures as transplantation. The concept is simple: A hospital and its specialists contract with an HMO or capitated group practice to care for patients with a specific chronic condition, such as AIDS, spinal cord injury, or congestive heart failure. In most situations, chronic care capitation is paid on a patient-by-patient basis. The fixed monthly payments vary by the patients' severity of illness. For example, the capitation payment for AIDS patients may be adjusted according to the patient's T-cell count.

The appeal of this market niche is limited to hospitals that have the specialized expertise to cost-effectively manage such chronic care patients. Success under capitation depends upon the ability of the hospital and collaborating physicians to lower hospital use and reduce customary stays, often substituting other lower-cost settings or ambulatory treatment. Diabetes treatment patterns, for instance, may vary 15 to 30 percent, measured by admissions and patient days.

Specialized services and settings present additional opportunities for chronic care subcapitation. Subacute care, for example, is the fastest-growing segment of the long-term care market, although the subacute care market is "not for the fainthearted" (Dunn 1996). Subacute services have current market revenues of $600 million, with forecasts by market analysts of up to $10 billion by the year 2000.

Hospice care is another growth market for subcapitation. Demand for hospice care is expected to double by the year 2000 (Montague 1996). Hospice care is both more appealing to patients than traditional terminal care and lower in cost. Almost 300,000 patients received hospice services in 1995, a number predicted to grow to over 500,000 patients by the end of the decade. Some 86 percent of hospice providers are nonprofit, but a number of forprofit firms are now entering the market.

Chronic care capitation is a risk-assumption arrangement that demands cost-effective care management. Hospitals considering this strategy must have full cooperation from physicians, including development of treatment protocols, continuous care management, aggressive substitution of lower levels of care, and scientific assessment of patient outcomes. Successful hospitals may be able to corner the market for their chronic care specialty, on a local and regional basis, with capitation subcontracts from a number of HMOs, integrated delivery systems, and at-risk physician organizations.

Strategy 5. Medicare Risk Contracting

Medicare risk contracting may be the most important—and potentially profitable—strategy for U.S. hospitals and physicians, given their high dependency on Medicare patients. Political pressures for a middle-class tax cut and reduction of the federal budget deficit may tempt Congress to think of Medicare as a "piggy-bank" for reforms (Toner 1994). The result is likely to be increased reliance by the Health Care Financing Administration on managed care strategies to put more Medicare enrollees into risk-contract HMOs.

But Medicare risk contracting so far has been concentrated in high-cost markets where Medicare HMO payments are higher. Payments can reach almost $600 PMPM, but Medicare HMOs can still lose money. In Minnesota, with heavy Medicare HMO enrollment, the Medica Primary plan earned a $4.9 million surplus, while competing Group Health lost $5.5 million on its two Medicare plans (Advisory Board Company 1994).

The Advisory Board Company stated that Medicare risk contracts are potentially the single most lucrative segment of capitated business (and may be the only way to protect all-important Medicare revenues). This is a huge potential market. Some 33 million Medicare patients could have signed up with Medicare HMOs, but only 4.5 percent did so. While the financial feasibility of Medicare risk contracting varies dramatically, due to differing levels of HCFA payments, it is possible for the arrangement to be profitable in most parts of the country. Medicare HMOs are still operating under a handicap—the "95 percent" payment limit for HMOs based on local Medicare health costs. The formula for setting Medicare HMO rates is complicated, with reimbursement that varies almost 100 percent from one region to another (see Fig. 4.3).

Five Stages of Managed Care

Figure 4.3 Medicare Risk Payments by Location

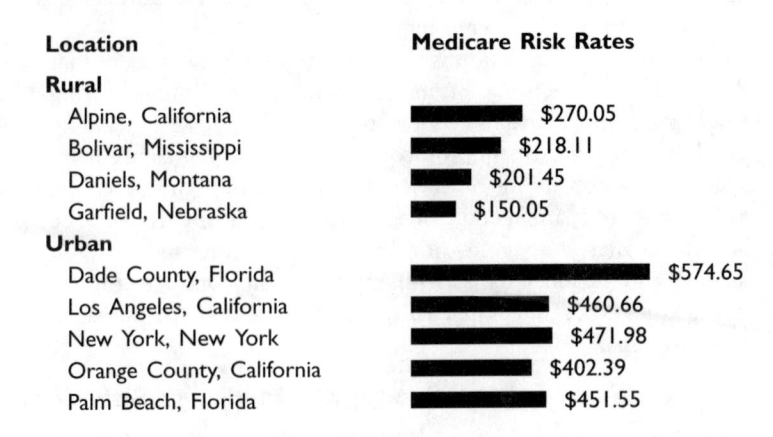

Location	Medicare Risk Rates
Rural	
Alpine, California	$270.05
Bolivar, Mississippi	$218.11
Daniels, Montana	$201.45
Garfield, Nebraska	$150.05
Urban	
Dade County, Florida	$574.65
Los Angeles, California	$460.66
New York, New York	$471.98
Orange County, California	$402.39
Palm Beach, Florida	$451.55

Source: Health Care Financing Administration; cited in "Capitation Strategies," Advisory Board Company, Washington, D.C., 1994, pp. 320–21.

Hospitals cannot afford to stay out of Medicare risk contracting. Medicare patients represent a significant percentage of hospital discharges and inpatient revenue. Medicare HMO capitation can generate substantial cash flow. Each Medicare enrollee may be worth three to four times the revenue in monthly premium, compared with under-65 commercial HMO enrollees.

Strategy 6. Partnership Capitation

In a partnership capitation strategy, a hospital and select members of the medical staff join together to accept full-risk capitation from payers. The purchasers may be HMOs, insurance companies, or self-insured employers engaging in direct contracting. The contracting function is provided by a jointly-owned management service organization or physician-hospital organization that represents all providers in the network. The partnership model is simpler to organize and can be started in a fraction of the time it would take to build a hospital-owned (or physician-owned) network.

A partnership capitation strategy enables the hospital and physicians to control 75 to 85 percent of the premium dollar, taking full responsibility for all patient care activities. In general, roughly 20 percent of the premium will be allocated for HMO administration and profits, 27 percent for hospital inpatient services, 13 percent for primary care, 26 percent for specialty care, and 14 percent for outpatient and ancillary services. Converting enrollees of a hospital's preferred provider organization, or capitating the hospital's employee health plan, can provide a base of covered lives. The hospital and physician partners may want to get an HMO license, or purchase a part or controlling interest in an HMO.

For a partnership strategy to work, there must be a physician-hospital organization to take on the contract and manage both patients and costs. Not all physicians will be willing to participate in full-risk contracting. Physicians interested in capitation should be organized in a subpanel. Better yet, the physicians themselves should organize, as a closed panel, with defined qualifications and periodic performance appraisal. To manage patients under capitation, the PHO will need a medical director, experienced managed care staff, and expert consultants. A data system must link all providers, with the capacity to generate the reports demanded by purchasers. Sufficient working capital must be available up front to cover the cash flow of provider payments. Arrangements for reinsurance will cover high-cost cases. Utilization management and quality assurance can be developed internally, or "rented" from an HMO or third-party review organization. It is essential to withhold a percentage of physician and hospital payments to build reserves for unforeseen costs and for future expansion.

Strategy 7. Network Capitation

When providers consider network capitation, they should think in terms of the region or state. Developing an at-risk network for provider capitation is among the best sustainable strategies for a managed care market, and the key to success is geographic coverage and the ability to offer choice of hospitals and physicians. A regionally distributed network of providers gives purchasers what they want—"pins in the map"—offering broad choice and easy access for consumers. Better yet, the network should incorporate the region's best-known and highest quality hospitals.

Some networks will be organized on the hub-and-spoke model, with high-visibility regional medical centers. Opinions vary with regard to membership of academic medical centers. Maryland has two statewide networks. One is Johns Hopkins University Hospital, one of the country's premier hospitals. The other network deliberately chose to have no high-cost tertiary hub, believing that purchasers wanted lower costs (Kenkel 1994).

A capitated network is a voluntary business arrangement, not a merger or acquisition. Thus a contractual network can be formed much faster than hospitals can be merged or physicians can be acquired. Each hospital brings its physician organization, organized as an MSO or PHO. A regional or statewide network MSO can contract on behalf of all physicians and hospitals, an excellent strategy for contracting with state Medicaid reform initiatives. Network organization positions hospitals and doctors to cut a "master deal" for exclusive provider contracting on a regional or statewide basis. Providers organized in networks can bargain from strength, overcoming the weaknesses of spot-market contracting, and uniting doctors with their hospitals to bargain together with HMOs, insurers, and employers.

Strategy 8. System Capitation

System capitation moves an integrated delivery system into full-risk arrangements with HMOs, insurers, or self-funded employers. The IDS is the source for all provider services, including hospitalization, medical care, and all other diagnostic or treatment services. Specialty services not available in the system (e.g., transplants) can be subcapitated to outside providers. In this model, vertically integrated systems take advantage of their own physician networks. Physicians and hospitals are part of a unified organization. They share a bottom line, they exercise discipline in clinical resource management, and they get preferential treatment from HMOs and managed care buyers. Some IDSs will own HMOs or insurance companies.

The goal of system capitation is *integration*—the disciplined management of capitation premiums. The winners are those integrated systems that reduce costs to live within limited capitation payments. Losers have two ways to fail: (1) they get a capitation contract but cannot control their costs; or (2) they are never even offered capitation and are passed over by HMOs, insurers, and direct-contracting employers.

System capitation and mergers between providers and HMOs or insurers are blurring the boundaries between payers and providers. HMOs are becoming integrated systems and acquiring primary care physicians, while hospitals and doctors are simultaneously starting provider-sponsored HMOs. There are multiple models for an IDS: (1) a hospital system owns physicians, (2) a physician organization owns hospitals, (3) a hospital system and physician organization merge or become partners in an exclusive relationship with no termination clause (e.g., Kaiser), or (4) an HMO or insurer owns or merges with a hospital system and physician organization. The strategic goal of the system strategy for capitation is the absolute merging of physicians and hospitals, preferably with a financing mechanism such as an HMO. With complete commitment by all parties, the system capitation strategy may be the most integrated of all models for managing capitation.

LOOKING FORWARD: NEW APPROACHES FOR CAPITATION MANAGEMENT

Capitation is expanding and maturing, creating new market opportunities for well-integrated physician groups and health systems. Primary care capitation, which was often introduced in Stage 2 and Stage 3 markets, is giving way to a new array of at-risk arrangements that focus on big-ticket specialty care expenditures and sharing risk with regional delivery systems.

Subspecialty Capitation

Primary care gatekeepers are far from obsolete, but a growing number of HMOs are turning to capitation for management of specialty medical costs. Capitation now accounts for 25 percent of HMO payments to medical subspecialists (Hamer 1996; see Table 4.2). Physician supply—and surplus—is a factor in such capitation. Psychiatrists are most likely to be capitated (41 percent), followed by radiologists (28 percent), and pathologists (28 percent). Emergency physicians were most likely still to be paid on a fee-for-service basis (63 percent). Almost half (46 percent) of physician payments by group-model HMOs are under capitation.

Formation of single-specialty physician groups for capitation got a boost from the federal government in 1995 when the Justice Department gave a favorable antitrust ruling to a proposed physician network that would have included 100 percent of the 85 board-certified dermatologists in South Carolina (Burda 1996). The Justice Department accepted the argument that the dermatologists would account for no more than 30 percent of the common skin treatments in any local market. Of the 23 integrated networks reviewed by the Justice Department and the Federal Trade Commission (FTC) since the fall of 1993, some 19 arrangements have received antitrust clearance. Physician networks must demonstrate that they share financial risk and are integrated as a single economic unit.

Access Management

Access management systems control costs and manage care beginning at the point of entry to the system—a telephone contact from an enrollee. HMOs, insurers, and capitated health systems

Table 4.2
HMO Reimbursement Methods for Physician Specialists (fee-for-service, capitation, relative value scale, salary)

Specialty	FFS	Capitation	RVS	Salary
Allergy/immunology	56%	27%	14%	3%
Anesthesia	56	27	14	3
Cardiology	62	20	15	2
Dermatology	56	26	15	3
Emergency medicine	63	21	13	3
Endocrinology	59	23	16	2
Gastroenterology	57	25	15	3
General surgery	58	24	16	2
Hematology/oncology	59	24	16	1
Infectious disease	58	23	16	3
Nephrology	60	23	16	1
Neurology	58	23	17	2
Neurosurgery	60	22	17	1
Obstetrics/gynecology	56	24	16	4
Ophthalmology	56	27	15	2
Orthopedics	57	26	16	1
Otolaryngology	57	25	16	2
Pathology	57	28	14	1
Plastic/reconstructive surgery	59	24	15	2
Psychiatry	46	41	11	2
Pulmonary medicine	57	24	17	2
Radiology	56	28	13	3
Rheumatology	59	22	17	2
Thoracic surgery	58	24	17	1
Urology	57	25	16	2

Source: Hamer, R. 1996. "HMO Industry Report." InterStudy Competitive Edge. InterStudy Publications, Bloomington, MN.

are creating toll-free telephone triage services to channel service demand and direct consumers to the most appropriate provider. Companies like Access Health of Rancho Cordova, California, are experiencing rising interest in their "access care manager" and "health link" programs, which dispense health advice, arrange for medical appointments, and provide care management to chronically ill patients.

Most access management services are optional—offered on a "value-added" basis by the HMO or capitated provider network to reduce consumer hassles and improve access to the health system.

Access management systems can also provide continuing care coordination for chronically ill populations, with conditions such as cancer, heart disease, and diabetes. In the future, tightly managed plans may use access managers as a mandatory "tollgate" to the system. All enrollees would be required to obtain prior approval from the access manager before scheduling an appointment or hospitalization or receiving emergency treatment.

Incentives/Risk Pools

Risk-pool arrangements are among capitation's most effective mechanisms for driving costs and use rates downwards. Incentive funds can be directed toward multiple targets:

- hospital costs (admissions, patient days, cost per case);
- surgical procedures;
- emergency medical services;
- ancillary costs (laboratory, radiology);
- referrals to specialists, or the costs of specialty care; and
- primary care (the percentage of patient encounters handled by primary care physicians).

Incentive capitation arrangements are becoming more sophisticated. In addition to volume and cost reductions, progressive capitation incentives are now focusing on qualitative factors, such as patient satisfaction, consumer complaints, HEDIS-type indicators (e.g., percentage of immunizations, Pap smears, mammograms), and disenrollment rates. Rewarding providers for promoting enrollment suggests that incentives may be reaching a more advanced level, adding longer-term goals such as customer retention to the short-term goals of cost cutting and profitability.

HMOs have identified disenrollment as a major cost of doing business. It is a problem both in high-growth markets like Dallas and Atlanta, where competitors are slashing prices to lure thousands of enrollees to switch plans, and in mature markets like San Diego and Minneapolis–St. Paul. In mature markets, HMOs are competing with expanded benefits and broader provider networks, which drive costs up. For plans with high disenrollment, the cost of acquiring additional enrollees may exceed the HMO's entire profit margin. Sophisticated risk-pool arrangements in advanced managed care markets like California are now refocusing goals away from cost reduction toward quality indicators and disenrollment and reenrollment.

Supernetworks

Regional provider networks and HMOs are edging toward capitation mega-deals. These large-dollar transactions will involve hundreds of thousands of covered lives in major metropolitan areas and even states. Providers are scrambling to develop super-PHOs for this potential market opportunity. In Baltimore, the Johns Hopkins HealthCare System linked with Louisville, Kentucky–based Humana, Inc. (Rudd 1996). The goal of this supernetwork is to market managed care across a region that includes Maryland, Delaware, Pennsylvania, Virginia, West Virginia, and Washington, D.C. Humana saw an opportunity to use the Johns Hopkins reputation to build membership away from its Washington, D.C. base. For Johns Hopkins, the network alignment was a means to channel patients into Hopkins-sponsored networks in pediatrics and oncology and to drive Humana's tertiary care patients into the Baltimore medical center.

Network capitation is the dream of many of the country's 3,000 physician-hospital organizations, but the early results of PHO development are disappointing—few contracts and little integration. PHOs have signed up relatively few HMO patients, and most PHOs have not evolved into fully integrated delivery systems (Jaklevic 1995). Hospitals are now recognizing the need to link their PHOs to form regional contracting networks. In Chicago, several Catholic healthcare organizations—Loyola University Medical Center, Resurrection Health Care Corp., Saint Bernard Hospital, Saint Francis Hospital of Evanston, Saint James Hospital in Chicago Heights, and Saint Mary of Nazareth HealthCare Network—have formed a joint venture, United HealthCare Network. Together, these hospitals and health systems intend to be one of the dominant managed care networks in the region.

STRATEGIES FOR PROVIDERS, HMOs, AND SUPPLIERS

Providers

Healthcare providers need to get organized for capitation, and fast. Hospitals should employ new capitation-oriented strategies quickly to avoid becoming commodities. They must invest in the development of physician networks, care management systems, and managed care organizations. Hospitals that create regional physician-hospital networks may have more bargaining power for exclusive agreements with HMOs and insurers. In the interim, the best a freestanding hospital may do is to pursue "niche" strategies until its managed care strategies and physician investments pay off with capitated enrollees.

Providers must adopt a managed care mindset. Hospitals should aggressively assist the HMOs and capitated physician groups to reduce hospital admissions, in-hospital service costs, and length of stay. Lowering hospital use rates quickly is intended to reposition the hospital for a permanently lower utilization "floor." Getting to that floor rapidly will reduce the pain and costs of transition.

For that all-important Medicare market, there are three approaches that hospitals can pursue to engage in Medicare risk contracting: (1) own, hold an equity position in, or start an HMO that becomes certified by HCFA for Medicare risk contracting; (2) own or become a partner with a multispecialty physician group that is contracting with a Medicare HMO; and (3) subcontract or subcapitate for hospital services with a Medicare HMO. If there is no Medicare HMO in the hospital's market, it should start one or develop a partnership with an outside HMO that is already HCFA-certified.

HMOs

The future of capitation—and U.S. healthcare—may be determined by how willing HMOs are to share premiums with providers. Should HMOs capitate providers broadly, or continue the current pattern of discounts and controls? Health maintenance organizations would make a mistake to stay with third-party review and micromanagement of provider performance. No managed care strategy has been as effective as capitation in giving providers incentives to reduce healthcare costs. The issue is trust between buyer and seller, and control or cooperation as the basis of their relationship. HMOs that fail to capitate providers will only drive hospitals and doctors to establish competing HMOs.

Suppliers

In the short term, capitation may damage the provider-supplier relationship. The result of provider capitation will be to slash all variable costs and reduce utilization levels. The results could be a 15 to 30 percent cut in supply purchases in the next few years. Cuts could be even deeper in some discretionary categories such as surgical supplies and anesthesia gases. Suppliers and distributors must accommodate capitation and be willing to enter into capitated arrangements. Baxter is experimenting with capitated surgical supplies. Reductions in surgical supply costs will be shared between providers and suppliers. Integrated delivery networks complicate the provider-supplier relationship. Suppliers, pharmaceutical manufacturers, and equipment makers must now establish relations with the new integrated provider networks, which may lead to deal-making outside of group purchasing organizations. The result could dilute the purchasing power of GPOs and lead to consolidation of purchasing groups.

SOURCES

Advisory Board Company. 1994. *Capitation Strategies*. Washington, DC: The Governance Committee

Burda, D. 1996. "Docs Get Their Way." *Modern Healthcare* 26 (2): 40–45.

Cochrane, J. 1993. "Experience Pays Off: Facility Prospers with Capitated Contracts." *Integrated Healthcare Report* (September): 5–7.

Coile, Jr., R. C. 1994. "Capitation Strategies." *Hospital Strategy Report* 6 (12): 1–8.

Dunn, D. 1996. "Subacute Care Offers Opportunities to Reduce Costs, Maintain Quality." *QRC Advisor* 12 (10): 1–5.

Eckholm, E. "While Congress Remains Silent, Health Care Transforms Itself," *New York Times*, 18 December 1994, pp. 1, 22.

Hamer, R. 1996. "HMO Industry Report." *InterStudy Competitive Edge* 5 (2): 1–156.

———. 1995. "HMO Industry Report." *InterStudy Competitive Edge* 5 (1): 1–109.

Jaklevic, M. 1995. "PHOs Fall Short of Expectations" *Modern Healthcare* 25 (41): 77–82.

Kenkel, P. J. 1994. "Physician-Hospital Collaborations Increase, Work to Capture Managed Care Contracts." *Modern Healthcare* 24 (14): 59–65.

Montague, J. 1996. "Dying With Dignity." *Hospitals & Health Networks* 70 (13): 13.

Rudd, T. 1996. "Johns Hopkins, Humana Team to Build Maryland MCO Network." *Healthcare Systems Strategy Report* 13 (1): 5.

Stearns, S. C., B. L. Wolfe, D. A. Kindig. 1992. "Physician Response to Fee-for-Service and Capitation Payment." *Inquiry* (Winter): 416–25.

Toner, R. "Groups Rally to Fight Medicare Cuts," *New York Times*, 18 December 1994, p. 19.

CHAPTER 5

Integrated Delivery Networks: Providers Organize for Managed Care and Direct Contracting

The battle is going to be won, not with one hospital competing with another hospital, but with one health care business ecosystem that has an insurance vehicle, a primary care and physician vehicle, and by hospitals competing with others that have organized in a similar fashion.

David Anderson, KMPG–Peat Marwick (Melville 1993, 4)

CONSOLIDATION IS sweeping the health field, restructuring providers into large regional and statewide networks of hospitals and physicians organized to contract with HMOs and large purchaser coalitions. America's 5,500 community hospitals and 650,000 physicians are scrambling to get organized to increase market leverage in managed care negotiations. Providers are creating regional provider organizations with the capacity to take a capitated, risk-sharing contract under managed care and direct contracting.

Integrated delivery networks (IDNs) are a response to the market's need for regionally organized arrangements of hospitals and physicians who can contract jointly under a "single signature" with managed care buyers. Managed care is becoming the principal strategy of both public and private purchasers of healthcare.

In many markets, the consolidation of providers into two to three competing IDNs is nearly complete. Employers are feeding the rush to managed care as well. More than two-thirds of insured workers are in managed care plans, and HMO enrollment surged sharply in 1994, doubling its growth rate to 8 percent (Eckholm 1994). The shift of government-sponsored Medicare and Medicaid patients into managed care is another reason for creating IDNs. State-level reform initiatives are putting many state Medicaid programs out to bid, converting Medicaid beneficiaries to HMOs. More than a dozen states have switched to Medicaid capitation and managed care, and another 12 to 15 states are waiting for HCFA waivers to do the same.

STAGE 4 WAR TO CONTROL INTEGRATED DELIVERY NETWORKS

Sponsorship of IDNs may vary from region to region. But who will ultimately control the networks? Payers or providers? Potential network managers include HMOs and other insurers, hospitals, academic medical centers, for-profit companies, and medical groups or physician management corporations. Provider domination of healthcare networks is not guaranteed. If the contest were held today, insurance companies and HMOs would win.

Today, insurers "own" the networks because they control the enrollees. HMOs and insurer health plans "rent" providers. Hospitals and physicians are vendors to the insurers. But insurers may not hold their dominant position into the twenty-first century. When providers unite to form integrated healthcare networks, hospitals and physicians negotiate from a position of strength with payers.

U.S. healthcare is headed toward a Stage 4 market of network warfare. This scenario features a head-to-head battle between provider-sponsored networks and payer-dominated plans. HMOs and insurers have assembled provider panels—"rental networks"— but providers have little leverage in these insurer-dominated arrangements. If hospitals and doctors hope to gain real market leverage against HMOs and insurers, they need to work fast. David Anderson, a senior consultant with Chicago-based KMPG–Peat Marwick, urges healthcare leaders to create an atmosphere of urgency. "Imagine that everyone in your organization is standing on a burning train platform, and that changes in healthcare are a moving train. The train is leaving the station; it's not stopping" (Melville 1993).

The biggest threat to the future of IDNs may be from within. Bickering over board seats, physician fear of hospital control, and tensions between primary care physicians and specialists could

Organize for Managed Care and Direct Contracting

sandbag IDNs just as their market opportunity is emerging. Providers must remember the first rule of the pioneers: When circling the wagons, be sure to fire out!

ESSENTIAL COMPONENTS OF AN INTEGRATED DELIVERY NETWORK

Basically, an integrated delivery network is a coordinated group of providers working together. Together, network partners jointly provide services through an integrated continuum of care, with multiple levels of services and settings. The network is a regional distribution system, with primary care access points across the market area, and strategically located hospitals to provide needed secondary and tertiary care. Not all services or settings have to be owned by the partners. Some network participants may provide services under contract on an as-needed basis.

What does it take to be a managed care network? Market consultant Gerald McManis lists the essential activities and strategies necessary to become a successful integrator of healthcare:

- ability to assume and manage *capitation* contracts;
- capacity to assess, monitor, and improve the health of a *fixed population*;
- effective *patient management*, with treatment protocols to ensure appropriate care in the most cost-effective setting;
- ability to demonstrate *outcomes* of all services in all settings to determine the effect of a patient's total care—and its cost;
- supporting *information systems* to create computerized patient records;
- *incentives* for physicians to make cost-effective decisions with the best long-term effect on patients;
- business relationship to *share risk* with primary and specialty physicians and the health system; and
- health plan function necessary for *direct contracting* with payers. (McManis 1994)

PROVIDER-SPONSORED NETWORKS

Provider-sponsored networks (PSNs) could be every hospital administrator's and physician's dream: contracting for patients directly with employers and government without an intermediary, HMO, insurance plan, or third-party administrator. According to Tim Crimmins, M.D., chairman of the Minnesota Medical Association, "There is enormous interest in returning control back to provider groups." The PSN concept is also "relatively easy to implement. It doesn't require a lot of government regulation. It's all at the private level, and doesn't require a Clinton 1,300-page health reform plan" (Weissenstein 1995, 29).

Provider service networks emerged as a key component of the Republicans' 1995 Medicare reform plan, ultimately vetoed by President Bill Clinton. Introduced by Congressman Bill Thomas, chairman of the House Subcommittee on Health, the PSN concept carried the blessings of the American Hospital Association and American Medical Association. In the GOP legislation, PSNs would be certified by the Health Care Financing Administration to sign up Medicare beneficiaries for capitation, without an HMO license. The PSN proposal drew enormous support from community hospitals and physicians, but failed when the Republicans' omnibus budget deficit reform package was vetoed by the President. The American Hospital Association is reviving the PSN concept as stand-alone legislation in 1997 in hopes of gaining new market opportunities for provider-sponsored IDNs.

Even without federal enabling legislation, PSNs are an option in sophisticated managed care markets where buyers and sellers are cutting out the intermediary. Large self-funded employers and business coalitions want to contract with networks for capitated, comprehensive packages of health services. The PSN concept is simple. Major employers and local business coalitions contract directly with networks of hospitals and doctors, cutting out the HMOs and insurance intermediaries. Employers get lower health costs, consumers get access with fewer hassles, and providers get a larger share of the premium. PSNs are a win-win concept for everyone—except the HMOs and insurers.

For providers, PSNs offer managed care contracts without the costs or hassles. Components of the PSN concept include:

- network of hospitals and physicians;
- enrolled patient population;
- self-insured employer or business coalition;
- regional market coverage;
- purchaser-provider direct negotiation of benefit scope;
- capitated premium, putting providers at risk;
- provider-set reimbursement schedule;
- provider-managed utilization and cost infrastructure;
- stop-loss, reinsurance, and out-of-area coverage to limit provider risk;

- purchaser-established performance standards ("report card"); and
- purchaser-provider shared information system. (Coile 1995)

PROVIDERS COMPETE WITH HMOs

The PSN movement is providers' direct counterattack against managed care plans, after years of discounting and controls by HMOs and third-party intermediaries. Employers define the health benefits they want covered and negotiate the price. Providers hold and manage risk, delivering all needed healthcare and reporting outcomes to purchasers.

Is it realistic for providers to think they might win bidding wars with HMOs? Direct purchasing opportunities will rise or fall based on whether providers can reduce the 15 to 25 percent administrative costs routinely taken "off the top" by insurers, HMOs, and third parties. If PSNs can reduce overhead costs, including profit, to 8 to 10 percent of premium—outcompeting HMOs, whose administration and profit level averages 18 percent—this provider-sponsored revolution may succeed.

Savvy self-insured employers, business coalitions, and government health programs are the potential buyers. Doctors and hospitals are the sellers, organizing provider networks on a regional and statewide basis. Up for grabs are over 225 million consumers whose health benefits are currently managed by insurance plans, HMOs, and third parties. High-profit HMOs are drawing fire from dismayed employers and irate providers. Some HMOs had medical loss ratios—what the plans spend for medical care—below 70 percent in 1995. Purchasers are steamed at getting less than 70 cents of health benefits for every dollar of employer health spending.

PSNs will not become a national trend without a fight. Insurers and HMOs complain that providers are acting like insurance companies, but without the regulations or reserves. Managed care plans fear loss of market share and, worse yet, declining enrollment from private-sector employers, a traditionally lucrative business. The Health Insurance Association of America and the Group Health Association of America are vehemently opposed to PSNs and are lobbying hard in Washington to prevent unregulated providers from becoming competitors. State health insurance regulators are also opposed to the PSN concept, and a number of insurance commissioners have ruled that providers must obtain HMO or insurance licenses before engaging in direct contracting.

DIRECT CONTRACTING REVOLUTION IN THE LAND OF 10,000 HMOs

Healthcare's next revolution is starting in Minnesota's Twin Cities, birthplace of the HMO concept. In mid-1995, the region's influential large-employer coalition, the Business Health Care Action Group (BHCAG) put its HMOs on notice. Beginning in 1997, when its current contract expires with Health Partners, the employers group will contract directly with more than a dozen local networks of physicians and hospitals. HMOs can only participate as organizers of local networks. To avoid insurance regulations, the employers will start with a modified fee-for-service system that will approximate capitation. Under the plan, providers will be given a utilization rate and will be rewarded or penalized for coming in above or below the target (Weissenstein 1995).

Providers are rethinking plans to merge into mega-networks with HMOs. Minneapolis-based Fairview Health System put its affiliation discussions with Blue Cross on hold after the BHCAG announcement. Minnesota's Blue Cross/Blue Shield still hopes to contract with BHCAG, using its sophisticated information and data collection system as a network organizer for the employer group. But clearly, the HMOs will suffer a major market defeat in Minneapolis–St. Paul, arguably the most advanced managed care market in the country.

Despite lowering health costs to about 80 percent of comparable markets, Minnesota employers still are not satisfied. "Basically we have tried everything else and we still don't have the right incentives in the market," explains Steve Wetzell, BHCAG executive director (Weissenstein 1995, 28). As evidence of lack of competition, Wetzell points out that 70 percent of the area's population belongs to the three major HMOs: Allina Health System/Medica, Blue Cross and Blue Shield of Minnesota, and HealthPartners.

Direct contracting with the buyers' coalition will open a window of opportunity for Minnesota providers. BHCAG has already screened more than 15 provider groups and has collected performance data on quality, access, and service, which consumers will use in choosing their own local network. For providers, direct contracting is a low-cost alternative to forming their own HMOs. Obtaining an HMO license in Minnesota is burdensome because of high regulatory barriers and reserve requirements enacted after several HMOs failed in the 1970s. "We Minnesota hospitals cut our own throats with HMO regulation," explains Roger Green, senior vice president for marketing and planning at St. Paul's HealthEast system. "After hospitals got burned by the HMO failures in the 1970s, they lobbied for high reserves to protect provider payments in case of future HMO bankruptcies" (Green 1995).

PHOs ARE TRAINING WHEELS FOR IDN DIRECT CONTRACTING

The investment in developing physician-hospital organizations is about to pay off. Health systems and physician groups that have established PHOs are now well along on the IDN learning curve. A small but growing number of PHOs have established direct contracting relations with employers, now some 14 percent of PHO business, according to a national survey by Ernst & Young (Weissenstein 1995; see Fig. 5.1).

HMOs and insurers are viewing physician-hospital organizations with a mix of skepticism and acceptance. Some health

Figure 5.1 Who's Contracting with PHOs?

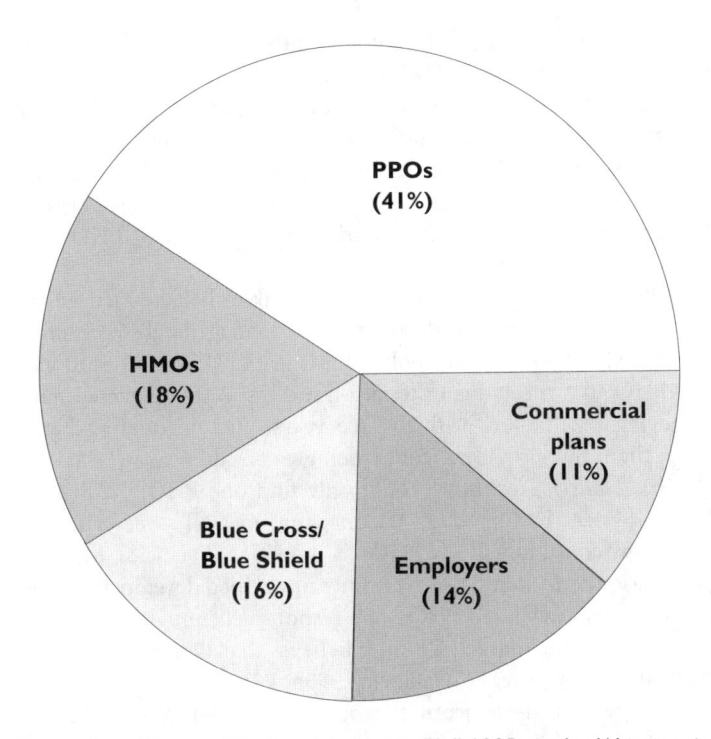

- PPOs (41%)
- HMOs (18%)
- Commercial plans (11%)
- Blue Cross/Blue Shield (16%)
- Employers (14%)

Source: Ernst & Young, "Physician-Hospital Profile," 1995; cited in Weissenstein, E. 1995. "Cut Out the Middleman." Modern Healthcare 25 (27): 29.

plans are welcoming PHOs as allies whose reputations may help in HMO marketing efforts. U.S. HealthCare's move into Maryland's highly competitive HMO market was buoyed by its affiliation with Johns Hopkins and its network of seven facilities. Other HMOs and insurance plans fear that network capitation could "train a competitor." Large, well-established PHOs may be considered as competitive threats by larger HMOs and insurance plans who prefer to control their own credentialing and quality. A survey by GHAA found that half of its HMO members perceive PHOs to be a competing form of managed care entity (Jaklevic 1995b). Providers hope to improve their contracting leverage by PHO and network formation. Many HMOs prefer to contract separately with doctors and hospitals, keeping providers divided and off balance, while HMOs drive tough bargains on physician fee schedules and hospital per diems.

UNTESTED PHOs MUST QUICKLY TIGHTEN UP FOR DIRECT CONTRACTING

Most of the nation's 3,000 physician-hospital organizations were set up to contract with HMOs. Now there may be new buyers: Medicare, Medicaid, large self-insured employers, and business coalitions. But PHOs are falling short of expectations. PHOs may be too understaffed and undercapitalized to be effective. A survey of 335 PHOs by the American Association of PHOs/Integrated Healthcare Delivery Systems found that 82 percent of PHOs had fewer than five employees (Jaklevic 1995b).

PHOs may not measure up as more than half-hearted efforts to save the status quo. California-based managed care consultant Nathan Kaufman is an outspoken PHO critic. He promises to visit any PHO that meets his criteria for success: 20,000 covered lives, achieving profitability within three years, and negotiating better rates than the providers could achieve on their own (Jaklevic 1995b). *Modern Healthcare* could only find one PHO, the Spectra Health System in Chandler, Arizona, that met all three criteria.

Many consultants view PHOs as transitional vehicles. Minneapolis-based consultant Daniel Zimmer has helped develop 30 PHOs, but questions whether PHOs are responsive enough to what is happening in the market. Zimmer believes that PHOs "may have a shelf-life of 3 to 5 years" (Jaklevic 1995b, 78). PHOs may not have the luxury of time to learn the business of managing care. The opportunity of direct contracting may push PHOs into full-risk capitation within a year.

A national survey by Ernst & Young (1994) showed that many PHOs were still in a formative state, and few had the capacity to manage large capitated populations (Jaklevic 1995b). Early signals on PHO development revealed that most were still emerging:

- Three in four PHOs were less than 24 months old.
- Leadership was recently arrived and inexperienced. More than 50 percent of PHO executives had been in place less than one year, and only 20 percent had prior managed care experience.
- Many PHOs had a medical director, but typically these physicians allocated less than 25 percent of their time to PHO affairs.
- In 75 percent of PHOs, physician panels were often specialist-dominated. Half of the medical panels were open-panel.

PHOs are beginning to win HMO contracts. Almost two in three PHOs had capitation contracts with HMOs, according to the Ernst & Young profile. Many PHOs had covered lives, but more than half had fewer than 25,000 enrollees. Some of these lives were likely to be hospital employees. More mature PHOs with at least 12,000 enrollees were more likely to have medical directors, utilization management programs, provider profiling capacity, and primary care case managers.

There is obviously much to be done, and quickly, if PHOs are to prepare for direct contracting with a wide array of purchasers. Staffing and leadership must be strengthened. Aggressive medical and cost management information systems must be put in place. Physician credentialing and networks must be tightened. Hospitals must cede contracting and utilization controls to the PHOs, and doctors need to align their medical groups and IPAs in close coordination with the PHO.

PHYSICIANS ARE SECRET WEAPONS IN MANAGED CARE STRATEGY

IDNs may have a secret weapon in the war with HMOs—active cooperation from physicians in managing utilization and costs under capitation. Provider-sponsored IDNs have a potential advantage of physician-hospital cooperation. HMOs make money by managing costs and reimbursement, not by delivering efficiencies in the process or outcomes of care. Care management in its current form might more accurately be called "care denial." Third-party review companies are paid on the basis of their denial rate, and HMO treatment guidelines are crude and negatively biased. There is little payer-provider cooperation.

On the other hand, physician-hospital cooperation is the foundation of IDN success. The real test of the IDN concept is whether doctors and their health systems can forge an alliance to manage patient care more effectively. Capitation forms the payment framework for collaboration. Physicians and hospitals share a risk pool as an incentive to reduce unnecessary utilization while protecting patients and outcomes. This level of cooperation does not come easily. Doctors and hospitals must bridge a chasm of mistrust if primary-sponsored networks are to be a win-win solution for providers.

At the Lovelace Clinic in Albuquerque, New Mexico, physicians are cooperating in a new episodes of care (EOC) approach to manage a patient's entire encounter with the healthcare system (Dearling 1995). Doctors at Lovelace have established 20 teams to develop EOC guidelines and clinical pathways. For example, Lovelace manages its diabetic patients through its primary care network, using a cooperative approach between specialist and primary care physician as specified in the EOC protocol. Primary care physicians are given disease-specific data on their performance in managing patients within the EOC guidelines. The protocol encourages patient involvement, with a Diabetes Care Card that tracks symptoms as well as system performance (e.g., did the physician check the patient's feet). As a result, the hospital admission rate for diabetic patients under the EOC program is only 2.3 percent, versus 4.8 percent in non-Lovelace patients, with inpatient stays of 5.2 days versus 7.2 days. Lovelace estimates it has saved some $1 million implementing nine EOC models (Weber 1996).

DISEASE MANAGEMENT TO CONTROL IDN COSTS

IDNs must aggressively develop standardized disease management like Lovelace's EOC protocols and clinical paths to manage the costs and outcomes of care. This strategy focuses on the medical care part of the premium. When an IDN assumes global capitation risk for all health services, its administrative costs must be low—less than 10 percent—for it to be competitive with HMOs and still earn a profit. Many buyers will place a 12 to 15 percent cap on administrative costs and profit. Managing the medical care part of the premium, some 85 percent of every health benefit dollar, must be the focus of IDN cost-management strategies.

The essence of physician-hospital cooperation lies in disease management. Mark Zitter (1994) defines "disease management" as a comprehensive, integrated approach to reimbursement, based

Organize for Managed Care and Direct Contracting

fundamentally on the natural course of a disease, with treatment designed to address the illness with maximum effectiveness and efficiency. Conceptually, disease management begins with prevention measures, well before the onset of acute illness. Programs define risk in an enrolled population, define and identify patients at risk, and institute preventive activities. When acute symptoms emerge, protocols direct the management of the illness in the most cost-effective way in the least-cost settings. Each patient's progress is routinely tracked, using outcome data captured from patient-completed surveys that query patients on the status of their health, functioning, and sense of well-being.

A number of health systems are pioneering the development of extensive disease management programs.

- Henry Ford Health System in Detroit, Michigan, has developed a provider-sponsored report card based on its Consortium Research on Indicators of System Performance (CRISP) system across a community-based system in a joint venture with the Mercy Health System of Farmington Hills, Michigan, and a dozen other large health systems like Allina Health System (Minneapolis, Minnesota), Baylor Health System (Dallas, Texas), Northwestern Healthcare Network (Chicago, Illinois), and Virginia Mason Medical Center (Seattle, Washington).
- Sentara Health Systems of Norfolk, Virginia, is piloting a sophisticated artificial intelligence–based computer program that uses predictive outcomes to provide clinical decision support.
- Dartmouth Medical School/Mary Hitchcock Health System in New Hampshire is implementing its COOP system for clinical improvement, using an inexpensive network of personal computers across multiple care sites.
- Advocate Health System in the northern Chicago suburbs has developed systems for tracking healthcare measures for specific diseases across its integrated delivery system.
- Graduate Health System in Philadelphia, Pennsylvania, is working with the University of Pennsylvania's CADU/CIS system, which uses algorithms developed by the Wharton School to risk-adjust and measure clinical outcomes.

POWERHOUSE IDNs ORGANIZE FOR MARKET LEVERAGE

The largest IDNs will be statewide, with dozens of hospitals and thousands of doctors. Very large IDNs are forming from New

England to California and across the Midwest. These IDNs are setting goals of managing 100,000 to 500,000 covered lives, under HMO contracts and from IDN-sponsored managed care products.

Regional IDNs are merging at the state level to increase market clout and attract statewide employers. In Arizona, two powerhouse systems have linked to launch HealthPartners of Arizona, which combines 2,400 beds, assets of $1.35 billion, and annual revenues of $1.3 billion (Shriver 1995). Phoenix-based Samaritan Health System, the largest multihospital system in the state, and Tucson-based Health Partners of Southern Arizona, the biggest IDN in southern Arizona, have linked their nonprofit organizations. The merger is "transparent to patients," says Samaritan spokesperson Beth Chasin (Shriver 1995, 17). Both companies retain their regional identities, but align managed care operations to serve 230,000 enrollees statewide in a jointly owned HMO.

Hundreds of regional IDNs are emerging. In New York, a Stage 3 market with 20 HMOs, the Mount Sinai Health System has expanded its regional network to 25 hospitals through two recent affiliations in northern New Jersey. Mount Sinai's network crosses state boundaries and religious sponsorship, adding three facilities operated by the Liberty HealthCare System in Jersey City and St. Elizabeth Hospital in Elizabeth, New Jersey.

MANAGEMENT SERVICE ORGANIZATIONS PROVIDE IDN INFRASTRUCTURE

Management service organizations are the cornerstones for developing integrated delivery networks. MSOs provide the governance structure and delivery network for HMO negotiations and direct employer contracting. They supply the management capacity and managed care contracting infrastructure, including finance, marketing, provider credentialing, network management, information systems, and customer service.

In the evolving concept of an IDN, the most important role of an MSO may be managed care contracting. Doug Goldstein of Medical Alliances defines an MSO as "a legal entity that provides administrative and practice management services to physicians, both individual physicians and/or group practices" (Goldstein, cited in Jaklevic 1995b). MSOs may be owned by hospitals, health systems, physician groups, and entrepreneurial investors. Most MSOs are subsidiaries that provide billing, physician profiling, credentialing, information systems, and utilization review. MSOs may acquire and manage physician practices. A number of MSOs are joint ventures between hospitals and physicians, although other partnerships involving HMOs, investors, and even employers are possible.

MSOs are highly flexible corporate entities for managed care and direct contracting. But are they working? They may disguise high costs and inefficiencies. Health Care Advisory Group's Steve Venable calls this possibility "a hospital hiding out in an MSO" (American Health Consultants 1995, 14).

Strategically managed MSOs should compete very effectively with HMOs as network organizers. In Ann Arbor, Michigan, a three-hospital joint venture, the Allegiance LLC (Limited Liability Corporation) assumed $150 million of risk and serves 105,000 capitated lives. Allegiance is sponsored by a three-hospital system owned by the Sisters of Mercy Health Corporation of Farmington Hills, Michigan. The four-year-old network has a number of HMO and preferred provider contracts, and Allegiance is now establishing an MSO to "house the tools of integration," and a future investment vehicle when there is a need for additional capital (American Health Consultants 1995, 14). The MSO will include management information systems, provider relations, and product development activities.

Managed care was the driving force in the creation of San Francisco–based California Pacific Medical Services. The organization is legally a combination of PHO and MSO, which includes four IPAs organized into a medical group. The PHO/MSO began in 1992 with the mergers of California Pacific Medical Center and Children's Hospital. Combined revenues flowing through the organization exceed $128 million per year, served by a PHO/MSO staff of 120 people. One of the reasons for this model's success was an early decision to keep the physicians in the medical group, and the administrators of the PHO/MSO, totally separate. "It was a brilliant decision," states Robert Branick, M.D., board chairman and executive director (American Health Consultants 1995, 15).

DEFINING THE ROLES OF IDNs, PHOs, AND MSOs

Confusion is widespread on the roles and status of IDNs, PHOs, and MSOs. Typically, the IDN is a regional joint venture of a number of hospital-sponsored PHOs. Most MSOs are subsidiaries of PHOs, although a regional MSO may be formed as an IDN service company to provide administrative and clinical management services. IDNs, PHOs, and MSOs provide new structures for developing managed care organizations. While IDNs are joint ventures today, an IDN might be the parent company for a future regional health delivery system.

Despite the fact that most IDN sponsors are not-for-profit hospitals, the Internal Revenue Service is skeptical about establishing IDNs as tax-exempt 501(c)(3) entities. Most of these provider-sponsored integration entities are considered taxable, either nonprofit taxable or for-profit corporations. The typical IDN, PHO, or MSO board is constructed with governance shared fifty-fifty with physicians and hospital representatives. But shared governance that does not reflect equity investment may cause legal problems for tax-exempt hospital and health system sponsors.

Creating a new legal entity provides an opportunity to create a new leadership model that balances hospital and physician interests. IDNs can develop small, corporate-style boards with market-motivated staffs. A few IDNs are adding "outside" directors, who may represent the community, major employers, or payers.

The underlying factor in IDN success may be leadership and governance. Governance consultant Jamie Orlikoff comments that, "While many organizations are now creating integrated structures designed to provide a seamless array of services, they are finding that structure, itself, is just the tip of the iceberg." Orlikoff believes the factors critical to IDN success are:

Outcomes measurement and management. Accurate and timely outcomes measurement facilitates continuous improvement of clinical quality and customer service.

Benchmarking. This involves identifying the best clinical service practices from a quality and cost perspective, and comparing performance with integrated systems in other markets.

Total Quality Management/Continuous Quality Improvement. This approach assumes that systems can always be improved in a process that is customer-driven and involves total participation across the organization, including physicians.

Leadership at all levels. Strong and enlightened leadership at all levels of the system must take charge, see the "big picture," and assume responsibility for all aspects of system performance.

Systems thinking. The various partners in the IDN must share the same values, assumptions, and vision that operate from the governance perspective of the system as a whole. (Totten and Orlikoff 1995)

IDNs WILL COMPETE ON QUALITY

IDNs will, of course, compete on price. It may be assumed that all major purchasers will demand lower premiums and health costs—all HMOs and insurers have to be competitive on price. But the ultimate purchasing criteria may be quality. Savvy self-funded employers are focusing on quality. In an independent survey of HMO quality and service CareData Reports found that one employer saved $500 per employee in healthcare costs by switching from low-quality to high-quality HMOs (Noble 1995).

Integrated delivery networks should exploit a real area of vulnerability for HMOs—customer ratings. CareData's study of HMO satisfaction in five major metropolitan areas found a range of customer satisfaction ratings from 36 percent to 69 percent. HMO enrollees were queried on 97 questions covering a wide range of qualitative and service issues. None of the more than 30 plans rated won a "highly satisfied" rating from more than 70 percent of its enrollees. Consumers told surveyors they were more likely to be satisfied by clinical quality than by the HMOs' customer service.

LEGAL STATUS: WHERE DOES THE IRS STAND ON IDNs?

IDNs, PHOs, and MSOs are pulling the country's largely nonprofit health organizations into the realm of for-profit entities. Even if their founders are nonprofit hospitals or health system 501(c)(3) corporations, IDNs, PHOs, and MSOs are not likely to be considered nonprofit or to qualify for tax-exempt status. The Internal Revenue Service generally considers these entities to be for-profit and taxable in nature, and warns further that hospitals and health systems may endanger their 501(c)(3) status if they provide all or a majority of the startup capital for these managed care entities. Healthcare legal advisors caution that IDNs, PHOs, and MSOs are joint ventures and that, where capitalization does not match governance, an IRS problem can develop.

Patrick O'Hare, a partner in the Washington, D.C. offices of McDermott, Will & Emery, outlines how nonprofit hospitals or health systems may protect its 501(c)(3) tax-exempt status while forming an IDN or PHO:

- Hospitals can structure financial support as a loan at market interest rates.
- Hospitals can take a larger share of control, with certain approval powers built into the bylaws, reflecting the hospital's larger stake in the equity.
- Hospitals can argue that it was essential to form the IDN (or PHO or MSO) in order to retain patients and survive under managed care, because loss of patients to managed

care organizations could jeopardize its survival as a charitable entity. (American Health Consultants 1995, 20)

PHYSICIAN MANAGEMENT CORPORATIONS POSITION FOR CONTROL OF IDNs

Physician management corporations are critical in the direct-contracting movement. PMC strategy is based on the "West Coast" model, which utilizes large multisite physician organizations as the lead agents in global capitation arrangements. Caremark International, the former subsidiary of Baxter Healthcare, and Nashville-based PhyCor, which merged with Med-Partners of Birmingham, Alabama, are among the nation's largest PMCs, acquiring dozens of physician groups and thousands of doctors in the past few years. Caremark/MedPartners' 7,000 physicians in southern California include doctors from Cigna Healthcare's staff-model physician network of 29 clinics, located across southern California from Los Angeles to San Bernardino (Jaklevic 1995a).

Increasing numbers of physicians are willing to become employees. Recruiting physicians is easier in an environment of managed care and declining incomes for many specialties. Medical groups, hospitals, and health systems have been aggressively purchasing physicians in the past three years, but the trend may be slowing. Physician recruiting firms report that starting salaries are declining, as more doctors choose security over independence. Financial offers to most specialists—even in some primary care categories—are falling:

- family practice: $129,000, down 2%;
- internal medicine: $130,000, down 4%;
- pediatrics: $120,000, up 9%;
- obstetrics/gynecology: $193,000, up 2%;
- orthopedic surgery: $242,000, down 8%;
- general surgery: $169,000, up 2%;
- cardiology: $182,000, down 2%; and
- psychiatry: $139,000, down 1%. (Droste 1995)

Physician-sponsored HMOs are gaining doctors' support—and their capital. Across the United States, with encouragement from the American Medical Association, state and local medical societies are coming together to create managed care plans. As reported by Bruce Japsen in 1995 in *Modern Healthcare*, in Florida, two physician organizations launched a campaign to raise $30 million to establish a statewide HMO. Under the name of Doctors Health Plan, the stock will be offered to the 17,000 members of the Florida Medical Association and the 3,000 members of the state osteopathic association. Sponsors hope to bring the HMO to market and begin enrollment in early 1997.

ACADEMIC MEDICAL CENTERS SEEK PARTNERS IN HUB-AND-SPOKE MODELS

Academic medical centers are reaching out to create hub-and-spoke networks to channel specialty referrals into the university while harnessing the market leverage and prestige of the university in managed care contracting. Some universities are developing HMOs to strengthen their managed care position. The University of Michigan and Cornell University/New York Hospital are among several academic centers that are moving into HMO competition with their own managed care products. In a search process like the one many other academic medical centers are now pursuing, the University of Missouri strongly considered affiliation or joint venture management in 1995. Eight potential partners responded to the University's request for proposal. Three final bidders were for-profit hospital management companies, including Tenet Healthcare, based in Dallas, Texas, plus a consortium of four nonprofit systems. Tenet, which operates three other facilities in Missouri, proposed creating a statewide feeder network for the University. In Columbia, the Missouri state capital, the proposal would align Tenet's Columbia Regional Hospital into the university's local orbit, giving the two hospitals leverage over the Boone Hospital Center, a 263-bed facility owned by statewide rival Barnes-Jewish-Christian Health System. Ultimately, the university chose to remain unaffiliated, but it will continue actively reviewing its options.

Restructuring academic centers for managed care will not be easy. The experience of the 554-bed University of Minnesota Hospital is a sobering lesson in what can happen if an academic center leaves its fortunes to the mercy of the managed care food chain (Scott 1995). Because the University's obstetrical unit dipped below 400 births per year, too few to support a teaching program, the university was forced into a partnership with Minneapolis-based Fairview Health Systems, relocating the program to Fairview's Riverside Medical Center. The university also moved neonatal intensive care units to Riverside. After aggressive cost cutting, the university had a bottom line of $11 million in 1994, following losses in 1992 and 1993. The university merged with Fairview, as regional consolidation forced it to abandon its "Switzerland" market stance.

LOOKING FORWARD: WINNERS, LOSERS, AND NO MIDDLE GROUND IN THE NETWORKING GAME

The shift to managed care and capitation is a win-lose game. Hospitals and doctors joined in a network will strengthen their negotiating power with HMOs and insurers, but still get lower payments. Payers will stabilize and control their costs of care under capitation but will lose power if they delegate cost management to capitated providers. Everyone must give up something if networks are to be integrators of care.

Hospitals will win or lose the war to become network organizers based on their ability to: (1) integrate clinical care services for efficiency, and (2) reduce the hospital share of the provider dollar. Reducing the hospital share of the capitation dollar is particularly important. Today, hospitals still get about 40 cents of every dollar spent on health services. That will shrink to 30 to 32 cents per dollar under capitation and managed care. But as IDN organizers, hospitals will share in the risk-pool savings with their physician partners.

Under capitation, the use of acute care hospital beds could be reduced by at least 25 percent over the next several years or sooner. Hospitals that are network organizers will themselves instigate the reduction of the hospital component. They must. Otherwise, there will not be enough money under capitated payments for the network to provide the full spectrum of services. Hospital care is the most expensive treatment option. Every other service is cheaper. The network will allocate patients to more cost-effective settings. That will inevitably reduce demand for acute care hospital beds. Hospitals as network organizers must understand this imperative and manage for efficiency.

Under capitation, the empty bed in tomorrow's hospital will be a sign of success, not failure—a complete reversal of today's administrative viewpoint. The incentives of capitation are fundamentally different. Healthcare executives who understand this must prepare their boards, medical staffs, and employees. There will be growth, but across the continuum of care. Capitation and managed competition will create the regional integrated delivery networks of tomorrow.

STRATEGIES FOR PROVIDERS, HMOs, AND SUPPLIERS

Providers

Hospital and medical group executives have little time left for making network connections. The deadline is 18 to 24 months for solidifying provider linkages on a regional and statewide basis. In this period, the best hospitals and physicians in the most preferred locations will definitively create or join networks. Hospitals with weak financial situations, poor locations, and aging plants will be chosen last, as will second-tier physicians with high costs of care and an interventional bias. Some will find no partners.

HMOs

Payers must move quickly to form strong agreements with the best, most cost-efficient providers. Insurer-organized networks should evaluate hospital and physician relationships immediately, and look for providers with good cost-management levels, quality outcomes, and partnership attitudes. The key decisions are which hospital-based IDNs and physician groups should be chosen as strategic business allies. HMOs must make these decisions with dispatch, or the best hospitals and doctors will enter into other arrangements. The window of opportunity for insurer network development of strategic business relationships is the next 12 to 18 months.

Suppliers

The development of networks has thrown a monkey wrench into established relationships between major suppliers, distributors, and provider-sponsored group purchasing organizations. Networks are likely to split GPOs or force a bidding war for their purchasing business, as Barnes-Jewish-Christian did with Voluntary Hospitals of America and American Healthcare Systems in 1994. Suppliers, manufacturers, and distributors may need a new marketing subdivision to establish relationships with the estimated 500 to 750 regional networks now emerging.

SOURCES

American Health Consultants. 1995. "The Magical Mysterious MSO: The Sensation of 1995 or a Bust?" *PHO Update* 2 (2): 13–24.

Coile, Jr., R. C. 1995. "Provider-Sponsored Networks." *Health Trends* 8 (2): 1–8.

Dearling, G. 1995. "Patients and Primary Care Physicians Drive 'Episodes of Care' Approach." *Outcomes Measurement & Management* 6 (9): 3–5.

Droste, T. 1995. *Medical Network Strategy Report* 4 (8): 12.

Eckholm, E. "While Congress Remains Silent, Health Care Transforms Itself," *New York Times*, 11 January 1994, pp. A1, A16.

Green, R. 1995. Author conversation. St. Paul, MN, 11 October.

Jaklevic, M. 1995a. "Caremark to Buy Cigna's System in Los Angeles." *Modern Healthcare* 25 (40): 3.

———. 1995b. "PHOs Fall Short of Expectations." *Modern Healthcare* 25 (39): 77–82.

McManis, G. 1994. "The New Delivery and Financing Realities." *Hospitals & Health Networks* 68 (16): 33–42.

Melville, B. 1993. "Ambulatory Care Site a Vital Strategic Decision." *Health Care Competition Week* 10 (17): 1–4.

Noble, H. G. "Study Rates Health Plans in 5 Areas Around U.S.," *New York Times*, 30 October 1995, p. A11.

Scott, L. 1995. "University of Minnesota Hospital Weighs More Mergers with Rivals." *Modern Healthcare* 25 (40): 16.

Shriver, K. 1995. "Samaritan, HealthPartners, to Form Largest Arizona Network." *Modern Healthcare* 25 (40): 17.

Totten, M. K., and J. E. Orlikoff. 1995. "There's More to Systems than Creating the Structure. HDG Roundtable." *Health Governance Digest* (July): 3–4.

Weber, D. O. 1996. "Lovelace Health Systems Boost Quality Cost-Effectiveness by Managing Comprehensive 'Episodes of Care.' " *Strategies for Healthcare Excellence* 9 (7): 1–9.

Weissenstein, E. 1995. "Cut Out the Middleman." *Modern Healthcare* 25 (27): 28–30.

Zitter, M. 1994. "Disease Management: A New Approach to Health Care." *Medical Interface* 7 (8): 70–76.

CHAPTER 6

Primary Care Networks: Integrators of Care in IDNs

> *Acute inpatient care, the "core" business of hospitals, is now being rapidly displaced by the growing emphasis on primary care and wellness. Healthcare systems must reorganize to reflect this change, . . . breaking down the "silos" or vertical structures in which hospitals function to begin to manage healthcare delivery on a population basis.*
>
> Stephen M. Shortell (Southwick 1994, 2)

PRIMARY CARE networks are the integrators of care that will dominate tomorrow's integrated delivery systems. Primary care networks will be the regionally distributed front line of clinical care delivery and cost containment, managing enrolled populations of 100,000 to 500,000 and more. Sophisticated HMOs and insurers believe the formula for success in a managed care market is simple:

Primary Care + Capitation = Market Dominance

Hospital-sponsored development of primary care networks is widespread. A survey by Physician Strategies 2000 found that 90 percent of sampled hospitals had established primary care networks or management service organizations to acquire and manage physician practices (Wagner 1996). Capital investment can mount quickly. More than 50 percent of the hospitals had already spent more than $1 million on developing primary care

Five Stages of Managed Care

physician networks, and another 30 percent planned to spend at least $1 million in the coming year.

Capitation is restructuring providers, payments, and power. Primary care physicians are capitated for all primary care services and paid to be gatekeepers, controlling all referrals to specialists and authorizing any surgery or hospitalization. Capitation places an absolute limit on provider reimbursement, and impels primary care physicians to be prudent managers of their enrolled covered lives. Primary care groups with their own hospital can take on global capitation contracts, subcontracting for all specialist and hospital services. The new economics of capitation dramatically demonstrates the efficiency of a primary care network as the integrator of care (see Table 6.1).

The strategic emphasis on primary care as the integrating mechanism recognizes there is a shortage of PCPs and a surplus of specialists and hospitals. Hospitals and health systems, physician groups, and insurers are bidding against one another to purchase primary care practices and organize primary care networks. Health systems are paying up to $100 million for large primary care–based medical groups with thousands of covered lives.

Table 6.1
Use Rates and Expected Demand under Capitation (assuming an enrolled population of 270,000 commercial lives, 30,000 senior lives)

Service/Setting	Use Rates per Covered Lives	Expected Demand
Primary Care	Commercial = 1 PCP/2,000 lives	135 Physicians
	Senior = 1 PCP/900 lives	36 Physicians
	Total PCPs	171
Hospital	Commercial = 190 days/1,000	51,300 Patient Days
	Senior = 1,000 days/1,000	30,000 Patient Days
	Total Days	81,300
Skilled Nursing	Senior = 535 days/1,000	
	Total Days	16,050
Outpatient Surgeries	Commercial = 36 procedures/1,000	9,720 Procedures
	Senior = 110 procedures/1,000	3,300 Procedures
	Total Procedures	13,020

Source: Golembesky, H. E. 1994. "A Structured Perspective of Market Evolution." San Francisco: APM, Inc.

Integrated delivery networks may need to refocus on physician network development instead of owning hospitals. Southern California's UniHealth, based in Burbank, downsized its hospital network and sold some of its stock in PacifiCare, the 2-million-member HMO, to create a $100 million investment fund for purchasing medical groups (Shinkman 1995). Consultant Steve Valentine observes: "UniHealth is trying to be an integrated delivery system. But more importantly, they see the shifting of dollars to physicians and medical groups, and they're following that stream" (Shinkman 1995, 14). UniHealth has moved into northern California, where it owns no hospitals, to acquire key medical groups in Santa Rosa and San Jose. UniHealth CEO Terry Hartshorn confounds critics by continuing to move aggressively into new markets: "We are talking to medical groups in every major metropolitan area" (Shinkman 1995, 15).

DEFINING THE PRIMARY CARE PHYSICIAN

These days, who is a primary care physician? By definition of the American Medical Association, PCPs include physicians trained in the medical specialties of family and general practice, internal medicine, pediatrics, and obstetrics/gynecology. The emphasis of primary care physicians is the management of general health needs, including diagnosis and treatment of acute and chronic conditions. Primary care includes prevention and health promotion and is provided in the context of the family as well as the individual.

With the increasing specialization of medicine, today's primary care physician is usually an office-based practitioner whose practice is predominantly ambulatory care. In the future, primary care physicians may follow the trend of European medicine: PCPs will be community-based and specialists will be hospital-based. A growing number of PCPs no longer admit patients directly to hospitals, and few deliver babies.

Forecasting the Need for Primary Care Practitioners

It used to be that the ratio of primary care practitioners needed to serve a managed care population was a simple 1:2,000. That is, one PCP met the routine health needs of 2,000 consumers. The Mullikin Medical Group, operating a 400-doctor multisite medical group across southern California, recommends a range of 2,000 to 2,500 managed care enrollees per primary care physician

(Menkin 1994). Mullikin's actual ratio on a local basis depends on the number of physician extenders employed in a specific office. The age composition of enrolled population also affects how many patients can be managed by one primary care physician. A higher percentage of newborns, young children, or seniors will bring the number below the 2,000 enrollee level.

The Kaiser Permanente Medical Group, affiliated with the nation's largest staff-model HMO, employs 148 primary care physicians to serve 390,000 enrollees in San Diego (Menkin 1994). This is a ratio of 1 PCP per 2,635 health plan members, but Kaiser also employs 56 physician extenders, a ratio of .38 extenders per primary care doctor. Another HMO located in New York employs primary care physicians in a ratio of 2,200, near the middle of the range recommended by Mullikin.

Evanston, Illinois–based Sachs Group has a database model and software to predict the need for primary care physicians. The current competition for PCPs suggests that more specialized planning criteria are needed to estimate need and to locate optimally a network of primary care practitioners. The Sachs model uses some 20 criteria in selecting target populations for location of PCPs. It predicts the number and type of primary care visits for the defined local population, using data from the National Household Interview Survey, and identifies the likely number of households without a primary care physician, projecting the need for additional doctors in the community. The model even predicts how hard primary physicians will work and how many patients they can see.

Local demographic data are the ultimate predictors of the need for primary care physicians. How fast is each target community growing? What are the age composition, family size, and number of households with young children? How many mature families are there with older children? The answers are in the database, using the latest census information available. Estimates of demand for primary care are assessed against market analysis of physician supply, group practice location, and hospitals as well as other freestanding centers for ambulatory services. With acquisition prices of $50,000 to $100,000 and up for primary care physician practices, the cost benefit of a Sachs-type analysis of the primary care market is obvious.

ECONOMIC ARGUMENTS FOR PRIMARY CARE NETWORKS

There are clear long-term reasons why hospitals should build primary care networks: managed care contracting, gatekeeping, and developing a decentralized delivery network. But there are excellent short-term reasons as well: revenue growth, repeat customers, and profits in the fast-growing ambulatory care market. Primary care will be *the* most frequently used service in tomorrow's integrated delivery systems. In southern California, the Friendly Hills Medical Group reported that 65 percent of its clinic visits were to primary care physicians (Barton 1994).

Visits to PCPs are ambulatory care services, and there are sound economic arguments for prudent hospitals to expand in this area. First is the matter of *ambulatory growth versus inpatient decline*. Since the mid-1980s, ambulatory services have grown 200 percent, while inpatient days fell by 20 percent. Cost-containment approaches and new technology favor ambulatory substitution for high-cost inpatient care.

Second is *percentage of revenue*. The strategic importance of primary and ambulatory care has risen dramatically, as ambulatory care revenues doubled as a percentage of total hospital revenue in less than 10 years, from 13 percent in 1983 to 24 percent in 1991 (see Fig. 6.1).

Third is *revenue per visit*. Perhaps the best "do-it-now" reason for expanding primary care is that hospitals are making more money on ambulatory visits. Back in 1983, an inpatient day brought hospitals about $460 in revenues, compared with $90

Figure 6.1 Ambulatory Care as a Percentage of Hospital Revenues

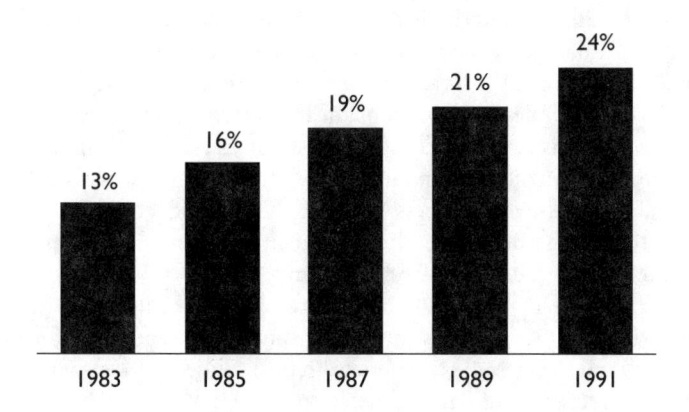

Year	Percentage
1983	13%
1985	16%
1987	19%
1989	21%
1991	24%

Source: Adapted from data by the American Hospital Association and Lammers + Gershon; cited in Melville, B. 1993. "Ambulatory Care Site a Vital Strategic Decision." Health Care Competition Week *10 (17): 1–4.*

for an ambulatory visit, a ratio of more than five outpatients to one inpatient. But by 1991, an inpatient day was worth $1,169 while an outpatient visit was worth $257. The ratio had improved to 4.5 outpatients to one inpatient.

Fourth is the *management of chronic illness*. Managing the chronically ill may be the best long-term reason for expanding primary care. Today, the elderly are healthcare providers' repeat customers. In the "age-wave" of the future, primary care gatekeepers and case managers will oversee the care—and manage the costs—of an increasingly elderly population (Melville 1993).

MEDICAID'S CAPITATED PHYSICIAN NETWORKS

With the collapse of national health reform proposals in Congress, state Medicaid contracting programs may provide the most effective solutions to the problems of access for the poor and uninsured. Medicaid reform projects will give primary care networks an opportunity to test their ability to manage millions of patients under a future of state-level health reforms.

Across the United States, a growing number of states are engaging in massive Medicaid contracting initiatives covering more than 5 million of the nation's 32 million Medicaid beneficiaries. Medicaid enrollment in managed care grew 57 percent in 1994, rising from 4.7 to 7.6 million Medicaid enrollees in fully and partially capitated health plans (Sardinha 1995). Arizona, Oregon, and Tennessee are among the states using a managed care approach to control rising Medicaid expenditures.

Contracting for hundreds of thousands of Medicaid enrollees will give primary care networks an opportunity to demonstrate their ability to control costs and manage utilization. The experience could be directly relevant to national health reform at a future time when Congress is again ready to address the nation's 40 million uninsured. If Medicaid capitation experiments are successful, this could encourage Congress to expand Medicaid coverage to uninsured groups such as children, pregnant women, and welfare recipients enrolled in "workfare" programs.

Primary care networks will be the front line of medical care in the growing number of states that are turning to managed care for their Medicaid beneficiaries. State-level reform initiatives appear to be the only remnants of national health reform, in which Medicaid enrollees may be pooled with the medically uninsured and state employees. The numbers could be large. Small employers and local government could also join these pools, increasing the number of covered lives to 15 to 25 percent of a state's entire population.

In California, for example, the state's Department of Health Services announced plans in March 1993 to shift to managed care as a major initiative to contain the growing costs of services to MediCal recipients (Frates 1994). California is giving first priority to converting MediCal beneficiaries into managed care enrollees in the state's most populous counties. A number of major California HMOs are participating.

Although prices were low, in the range of $65 to $85 per member per month, California's Medicaid managed care buyers anticipated that physician groups and health systems would compete hard to win a share of this 3-million-enrollee market. The California Department of Health Services used its own criteria to evaluate physician networks, including:

- quality comprehensive care;
- demonstrated concern for MediCal patients;
- ethnic diversity, linguistic capacity, and cultural sensitivity;
- geographic distribution of service providers;
- emphasis on prevention and health promotion;
- effective patient care management;
- primary care gatekeepers;
- care management system; and
- service guarantees for prompt treatment.

Can HMOs accustomed to treating the diseases of the middle class adapt to treating the health conditions of poverty? The MediCal capitation program recognizes the special needs and problems of serving a disadvantaged population. Provider networks must incorporate mechanisms to guarantee access, including locating physicians in areas of concentrated Medicaid population and providing transportation when needed. Providers must be culturally sensitive, such as providing a 24-hour bilingual "advice nurse" telephone triage service. California also seeks capitated networks that include "safety net" physicians already serving Medicaid patients, community health clinics, and disproportionate-share hospitals. This will mean that HMOs, insurers, and health systems seeking to compete for Medicaid contracts must develop provider relationships and service outlets directly in the areas to be served.

Whatever happens, this experience bears watching. California has one of the nation's largest Medicaid populations, covering about 10 percent of the state's population. The California strategy for converting MediCal to managed care has met with controversy since its announcement, specifically from public hospitals, who sought an exclusive arrangement. But the state is pressing forward with its plans to convert Medicaid enrollees to capitation in community networks. Medicaid contracting can provide an opportunity for providers and their HMO and insurer partners to develop integrated delivery systems for national health reform.

EIGHT MODELS FOR ORGANIZING PRIMARY CARE NETWORKS

In the rush to integration, there are a number of models to consider for organizing primary care practitioners. Some models are hospital-sponsored while others are physician-organized.

Model 1. Open-Panel Independent Practice Association

Many primary care networks are formed with an open-panel approach, accepting any willing physician who is currently licensed or board-certified in primary care. But these lightly structured organizations will gradually tighten their membership criteria and credentialing process to become closed-panel organizations. Open-panel IPAs are too unstructured to survive the shift to capitation. Stephen W. Hatch comments that "open PHOs are having trouble moving to selective panels—toward a more closed PHO form—because political will is lacking or the means to go through some kind of screening or selection process is not being developed" (Droste 1994).

An open-panel approach has worked to link physicians to insurers and HMOs on a fee-for-service basis. But more and more, payers are moving from discounts to capitation for physician payment, starting with primary care physicians. By moving to capitation, the HMOs hope to shift to physicians the risk and cost of managing costs and care. The move from open-panel to closed-panel must be systematic, however. Purists may want to limit the panel to specific physicians when creating PHOs, but "all hell can break loose" if doctors are arbitrarily left out of the organization, cautions Richard L. Riece, M.D., president of the National Association of Physician-Hospital Organizations (Droste 1994).

Model 2. Closed-Panel Physician-Hospital Organization

Capitation is the reason for creation of closed-panel primary care networks that monitor physician performance, establish clinical pathways, and work within a per member per month budget. Physician groups must demonstrate clinical and economic self-discipline under prenegotiated capitation rates, or they lose money.

Doctors are at risk, unless the hospital is willing to cover the losses—which is not a sustainable strategy. HMOs demand a distributed network of primary care physicians willing to take capitation payments to manage the routine health needs of their members.

Toughening up the medical network is an essential PHO task, if the providers are able to handle capitation. For example in suburban Indianapolis, 122-bed Riverview Hospital formed a 25-doctor primary care network in response to a demand by Methodist Hospital's HMO M Plan. Although M Plan members were only 400 of Riverview's 5,400 inpatients, Riverview saw the shift to capitation as inevitable. The HMO needed a minimum of 25 primary physicians in the capitated network by April 1, 1994, with agreement from Riverside's specialists to shift from fee-for-service to capitation when M Plan reached 10,000 enrollees.

To create the primary care network, Riverside formed a physician-hospital organization. Governance was fifty-fifty, with three primary care physicians and one specialist balancing two board members and two administrators. Specialists were skeptical, but 50 to 60 physicians of the hospital's 100-doctor medical staff have initially expressed interest in the PHO. Riverview is also discussing forming a super-PHO with the nine hospitals that make up the Suburban Hospital Group, an affiliation of Indianapolis-area facilities. The super-PHO could contract for the entire regional network of physicians and hospitals.

Model 3. Group Practice Without Walls

A group practice without walls is a form of medical group practice in which independent physicians form a loose alliance to share overhead costs and negotiate payer contracts. Doctors can establish these clinics without walls to operate with little or no hospital involvement, but some are hospital-sponsored or joint ventures with hospital or health system investment.

Primary care physicians are attracted to this model because it operates in a highly decentralized manner. Participating physicians are largely autonomous. The doctors manage their own offices, hire their own staff, see their own patients, and are reimbursed on a fee-for-service basis. Physicians share expenses but not revenues. There may be joint ownership of certain ancillary services. Primary care physicians who want to contract as a group to engage in capitation and risk management may use the without-walls concept to organize simply and inexpensively.

The group practice without walls may be one of the fastest, cheapest ways to develop a primary care network. On a long-term basis, though, it is probably a transitional strategy. The overhead costs are very high, because most participating practices are small and operate independently. For example, Sac-Sierra Medical Group of Sacramento, California, was one of the pioneering group practices without walls, organized in the mid-1980s to give its independent practitioners a contracting vehicle in the fast-growing managed care market. It affiliated with the Sutter Health System to gain capital for expansion. The group grew to 140 physicians but was facing losses of $6 million to $8 million when it decided to restructure as a primary care–based group in 1993, shrinking to 80 doctors with only 20 specialists (Golembesky 1994). The remaining doctors consolidated their practice sites and slashed overhead.

Model 4. Primary Care Division

Hospitals and health systems are building their own primary care divisions. In this arrangement, primary care physicians are hospital employees, part of a directly managed division of the system. The primary care division is generally built through physician acquisition and is often managed by a physician executive. In practice, the division operates as if it were a multisite medical group, with its own physician advisory board for credentialing, medical policy, and physician governance.

In Portland, Oregon, the Sisters of Providence Health System is developing a third-generation model for its heavily managed care marketplace (Southwick 1994). First-generation managed care plans discounted fees, while second-generation plans policed providers with severe restrictions on care. Third-generation managed care organizations focus on clinical integration and continuous quality improvement. Greg van Pelt, who chairs the clinical integration team, puts the new generation in perspective: "There is the concept of people belonging to a life plan of health as opposed to episodic intervention in their life." To focus on the consumer, the Sisters of Providence's new model is clinically driven, not financially driven.

Physicians in Providence's medical division were prominent in all discussions of management strategy and clinical integration. Developing a primary care network was a core strategy for the medical division of Providence's Oregon system. The ratio of specialists to primary care physicians was 4:1. Over time, the Sisters hope to move that closer to 2:1, and ultimately 1:1. In January 1993, the system formed a primary care division that employed 65 physicians. The specialists' dominance was being reduced as the system recruited primary care physicians, but the imbalance persisted for some time because of the dearth of primary care doctors being trained.

Creating a primary care physician network may be the second-most important strategy for survival in a managed care era, according to Patrick Hays, former executive of Sutter Health System: "Our focus is on continuing to grow our physician network, and then to build, acquire, or develop relationships with facilities as we need them (Cerne 1995). Sutter puts vertical integration with HMOs and physicians above horizontal integration with hospitals. Sutter's Sac-Sierra group practice without walls is only one part of the health system's strategy for physician development. By 1995, Sutter employed 478 doctors organized in five nonprofit foundations, backed up by 2,100 physicians in IPAs affiliated with the central California integrated delivery system.

Model 5. Primary Care–Based Multispecialty Group

Multispecialty physician groups can be a major market force in capitation contracting, but they must have a strong primary care base. Staff-model physician organizations are developing more flexible networks of community physicians to serve regional markets. Albuquerque's Lovelace Clinic is a case study in the development of a multispecialty clinic that has become a regional managed care plan. In the process, the clinic had to diversify its traditional emphasis on specialty medicine, developing a strong primary care orientation.

The Lovelace experience demonstrates the growing importance of primary care in the evolution of multispecialty clinics in a managed care marketplace. In 1976, this large multispecialty medical group had an excellent clinical reputation and owned a hospital. But Lovelace was losing patients and referrals, locked in market warfare with the specialty facilities owned by competitors Presbyterian Southwest and St. Joseph. The clinic had virtually no primary care physicians when it made a strategic decision to decentralize and build a network with family practitioners and urgent care centers.

Lovelace had to reorient itself from specialty care to primary care, and reach out to serve its customers. Within a decade, Lovelace had recovered strongly, thanks to its development of a primary care network. At the 1986 board retreat, the Lovelace CEO told the board, "We can survive the loss of the orthopedic department tomorrow, but we cannot survive the loss of the primary care departments!" (Schultz 1994). One of Lovelace's physician board members was even clearer, telling his colleagues, "Hire only family physicians." Lovelace is now affiliated with Cigna Insurance in a staff-model organization for the Albuquerque region and is the most integrated of the three dominant health systems.

Model 6. Ambulatory Care Satellites

Ambulatory care satellite clinics will be the primary care service centers for managed care providers. The St. Joseph Healthcare System in Albuquerque, New Mexico, has established such clinics, placing primary care physicians in "integrated service clusters" located around the Albuquerque market to serve St. Joseph's managed care enrollees (Barton 1994). More than 50 percent of Albuquerque residents are HMO members. Each cluster of physicians is an integrated group practice, owned by the healthcare system, with a majority of primary care physicians.

St. Joseph has organized the Medical Network of New Mexico (Med-Net) to provide a variety of contracting and affiliation opportunities for the medical staff of this three-hospital system. St. Joseph physicians may affiliate through the open-panel independent practice association, the closed-panel joint practice organization (JPO), or the hospital-owned integrated group practices, in a spectrum of integration alternatives. The system operates a Practice Resource Center to provide support services to physicians in the IPA and JPO. Med-Net capitates its primary care physicians and is moving its specialists toward capitation as well.

Med-Net is a model of the physician-friendly approach to building physician networks. It is designed from a concept of shared values and a team approach between the health system and physicians. Governance is shared, with physicians holding six of the nine seats on the board of directors. Ray Barton, the former St. Joseph CEO, describes the health system's approach as one of mutual trust and respect with "no fear tactics." There are multiple options and choices for physician integration, and shared risks and rewards between doctors and the healthcare system.

Academic medical centers are aggressively establishing primary care satellite networks. The teaching centers can no longer count on informal referral patterns to feed patients to their teaching programs. If they are to compete in a managed care marketplace, academic centers need to create their own regionally distributed network of primary care physicians.

For inner-city neighborhoods often underserved by health facilities, mission-driven hospitals like St. Mary's in Rochester, New York, have established networks of community-based primary care clinics. St. Mary's won the 1996 Foster G. McGaw Prize for excellence in community service (Larson 1996). As the first hospital in Rochester, it is the only health delivery system providing primary care at seven inner-city sites and 17 practices in local and suburban neighborhoods. Among its outreach initiatives, St. Mary's was cited for Healthreach, a lifestyle improvement program; Healthy Moms, for low-income pregnant women; and Healthcare for the Homeless People.

Model 7. Insurer-Owned Primary Care Network

Insurance companies, Blue Cross plans, and HMOs are recruiting and acquiring their own primary care physicians. Giant insurance companies and entrepreneurial HMOs are organizing PCPs into groups with practice locations strategically located across a market region. Prudential Healthcare System's Southern Group is moving aggressively to position the insurer as the HMO with its own primary physician network (Rudd 1994). Prudential has recruited 100 physicians to serve its enrollees in 10 cities across the South. For example, in Charlotte, North Carolina, Prudential-owned Carolina HealthCare Group expanded its 24-doctor group with 20 new PCPs in 1993. Prudential physicians will provide services for PruCare HMO and PruCare Plus point-of-service enrollees. Prudential enrollees constitute 90 percent of the insurer-owned medical groups' patients.

What attracts young physicians to sign up with an insurer? A definite appeal is the economic security of working for a medical group with guaranteed salaries and assured patient volume. Some physicians feel more independent—at least they are not working for a hospital. The insurer provides week-long management training for new physicians in managed care and coordinates recruitment efforts from its Atlanta regional headquarters. Doctors sign one-year contracts with Prudential, and turnover is low. Prudential's Health First Medical Group in Memphis, Tennessee, lost only 1 physician from its 45-doctor group last year, and recruited 10 more doctors.

Blue Cross plans are the latest insurers to adopt the staff model for delivering primary care through company-owned primary care clinics. In New Jersey, the Blue Cross and Blue Shield plan opened a statewide integrated delivery network of ten family health centers in 1995. The conversion of insurers like Aetna, Prudential, and Blue Cross to a staff model of physician employment—the abandonment of their traditional reliance on independent practitioners—may be one of the most important trends in the movement toward integrated delivery systems.

Model 8. Physician-Owned Management Service Organization

Physician-owned management service organizations are the foundation for doctor-driven healthcare delivery systems. They may be the antidote to hospital-owned MSOs, which are acquiring physician practices and putting doctors permanently in the hospital's orbit. In contrast, physician-owned MSOs give independent physicians and small medical groups a new vehicle for contracting with HMOs, insurance companies, and self-insured employers. In the future, they could be the physician components of regional delivery systems under national health reform.

MSOs may purchase and manage physician practices, and MSOs may be nonprofit or for-profit corporations. According to healthcare attorney Charles Bond, the advantages of a physician-sponsored MSO include:

- *Capital.* A for-profit MSO can raise capital from its member physicians, issue and sell stock, borrow from a bank, allow partial hospital investment, and seek venture capital.
- *Group purchasing.* The cost benefits of group purchasing alone can justify the creation of an MSO, even without other benefits (e.g., contracting).
- *Reduced overhead.* Consolidation of the business functions permits physicians to spend increased time with patients (increasing revenues), as well as lowering overhead by centralizing administration and "back-room" functions such as finance, billing, and insurance.
- *Collective contracting.* Where an MSO is coupled with an integrated medical group, it may collectively bargain for the doctors with HMOs, insurance companies, and employers.
- *Credentialing, quality, and efficiency.* Strong credentialing, quality assessment, and utilization review can be provided by the MSO, giving physicians more control over their practice patterns and costs.
- *Asset value.* Individual physician practices are worth relatively little, but collectively, as a medical practice integrated by an MSO, the equity potential of the group could be worth much more to a hospital, health system, or outside investor. (Coile 1994)

Primary care–focused physician MSOs may be constructed as a group practice without walls or a more integrated multisite group practice. The MSO concept is flexible. Physician ownership of the MSO is paramount. Physicians want to control their own economic destinies and collectively retain their professional autonomy (Bond 1994). Bond cautions doctors against "hitching their wagon" to a particular hospital, because HMOs and insurers may prefer other institutions. Physicians and hospitals should be linked by contract, not control, to maintain parity in the relationship. By attracting doctors who want their own contracting organization, the physician-owned MSO may provide a competitive alternative to hospital-sponsored MSOs or independent practice associations.

MSOs will manage regional and even statewide physician networks. In northern California, the powerful Hill Medical Group is a 1,200-physician IPA under the management service organization model (Pulley 1994). Hill contracts for about 170,000 prepaid capitation enrollees in the East Bay region. Hill also manages the IPAs of Catholic Healthcare West (CHW), a San Francisco–based system with 14 hospitals. CHW's business arrangement with Hill could be a major building block in the creation of a California-wide Catholic healthcare network.

ROLE OF NURSING IN THE PRIMARY CARE TEAM

The primary care practitioner a majority of Americans may see for routine health needs in the future could be a nurse. Cybernurse, telecommunicator, access manager, resource allocator, quality monitor, care coordinator, and hands-on therapist—these are a few of the roles nurses will play in the twenty-first century (Coile 1995). American healthcare is being radically reshaped by managed care, systems reengineering, competitive health policy, and cost-sensitive employers. Nursing is at the vortex of competing pressures for cost containment and quality improvement. Leah Curtin, editor of *Nursing Management,* predicts: "A number of experiments in health service delivery will be tried, but the only really successful ones will be those in which nurses remain at the heart of patient care delivery" (Curtin 1994).

Nurses, especially those with advanced clinical training, are well prepared for a number of primary care roles. Across settings, services, and even time zones, nurses will play a central role in the leadership and provision of all future primary care services. They may be:

- managing the gateways to the health system;
- centrally positioned as system controllers and care managers;
- closest-to-the-patient caregivers and health team leaders;
- clinical informatics specialists interpretating data;
- risk-managers for those with genetic and lifestyle health risks;
- behavioral modifiers who promote healthy habits;

- continuous care coordinators for frail and chronically ill patients; and
- community-based intervenors to mitigate health threats. (Coile 1995)

LOOKING FORWARD: A FEEDING FRENZY OF PRIMARY CARE NETWORKS

Creating primary care networks is reaching a "development frenzy," cautions Donald Schultz (1994), vice president of the Henry Ford Health System. PCNs are the front-line service system for thousands, even millions, of consumer covered lives, and HMOs, entrepreneurs, and hospitals across the nation are constructing them with a newfound fervor.

Primary care physicians' major contributions to integrated health systems are: (1) as access points for the network; (2) controlling costs under managed care and capitation; (3) as gatekeepers to specialty care and hospital treatment; (4) in occupational medicine; and (5) in consumer relations. The shortage of primary care physicians has prompted a bidding war to purchase primary-based physician practices, and salaries of $100,000 to $140,000 per year to recruit young graduates fresh from training.

Established primary care groups are fetching premium prices, commonly averaging $200,000 to $300,000 per physician, but rising to $1 million per doctor in some locations. Illinois-based Caremark, a former subsidiary of Baxter Healthcare, paid $140 million for the Friendly Hills Medical Group in southern California. Friendly Hills is a nationally prominent physician organization with extensive managed care and capitation expertise, and a 60:40 ratio of primary care physicians to specialists. The price of about $1 million per doctor included a hospital, a 140-physician group, and a community hospital.

The rapid shift to primary care has left many physician specialists feeling "out in the cold." Specialists know they will manage most of the high-cost patients under managed care, even under a gatekeeper model. Turf warfare threatens to open up major rifts between primary care doctors and medical subspecialists. The emerging conflict has led Doug McKell, president of Physician Strategies 2000, to ask, "Can—or should—primary care dominate the 'new' healthcare system?" (McKell 1994). McKell advises hospitals, health systems, medical groups, and insurers and HMOs to move as quickly as possible if they hope to establish a primary care network in a competitive marketplace. Specifically, McKell tells network organizers to:

- Create a critical mass of primary care physicians.
- Develop a financing organization (e.g., an HMO).
- Demand that physician leadership ignore naysayers.
- Coordinate primary care physicians' business marketing.
- Develop an integrated information management system.
- Discover primary care solutions that focus on patient care needs. (McKell 1994)

Is the bidding war for primary care practices over? Perhaps. Many U.S. hospitals have acquired primary care physicians and are now incurring losses from those hospital-owned practices. Reasons for the losses include: (1) the hospital lacked the infrastructure to manage medical groups; (2) the hospital paid too much for the practices; (3) the salary guarantees were too high; (4) the loss of economic incentives for physician productivity; and (5) the physicians adopted a nine-to-five attitude. On a long-term basis, a hospital may consider spinning off its primary care physicians into an independent for-profit medical group, with the hospital maintaining a strategic minority investment and seats on the board.

STRATEGIES FOR PROVIDERS, HMOs, AND SUPPLIERS

Providers

The shift to managed care and capitation places a premium on organizing primary care physicians. PCPs will be the gatekeepers and integrators of care for large groups of enrolled patients. The emphasis on primary care is raising tensions with specialists, whose authority and referrals are being challenged by primary care practitioners. Primary care networks are critical to building the integrated delivery networks of the future. At the same time, providers must head off the growing tensions between primary and subspecialty physicians. Sharing capitation is the best way to foster multispecialty cooperation.

HMOs

Managed care plans are recognizing the strategic role to be played by primary care, and actively building primary care networks through contracts and acquisitions. But the high prices being paid for primary care groups should arouse caution. Are hospitals, HMOs, and entrepreneurs going to bid up the value of PCPs beyond their ability to control costs or manage ambulatory care patients? HMOs should pursue a balanced strategy of physician development that encourages multispecialty collaboration for cost-effective care.

Suppliers

The rise of primary care physicians, and their key role as gatekeepers and resource managers, make it imperative for suppliers to open lines of communications to these decision makers. Primary care–based medical groups are becoming dominant in many integrated delivery networks. Suppliers need to involve primary care physicians actively in product development, marketing, pricing, and customer service activities.

SOURCES

Barton, R. 1994. *The Healthcare Market "Triad."* Albuquerque, NM: St. Joseph Healthcare System (unpublished).

Bond, C. 1994. "Strategic Use of MSOs." *Cincinnati Medicine* (Winter): 28–31.

Cerne, F. 1995. "Sutter Health: Innovative System Faces Up to Challenges on the Integration Speedway." *Hospitals & Health Networks* 68 (21): 56.

Coile, Jr., R. C. 1994. "The Leading Edge: Doctor-Owned MSOs and a Constitutional Convention." *Healthcare Forum Journal* (March/April): 86.

———. 1995. "Nursing 2000: Future of the Profession Under Competition, Capitation and Consolidation." *Journal of Advanced Practice Nursing* 1 (2): 21–26.

Curtin, L. L. 1994. "The Heart of Patient Care." *Nursing Management* 25 (5): 7–8.

Droste, T. M. 1994. "PHO Physician Panels: Inclusion or Exclusion?" *Medical Staff Strategy Report* 3 (4): 1–3.

Frates, J. 1994. "MediCal Managed Care: Issues for Capitated Physician Contractors." *Northern California Medicine* 5 (2): 20–21.

Golembesky, H. E. 1994. *Integrated Delivery Systems: Examples of Physician-Hospital Linkage Models.* San Francisco: APM, Inc.

Larson, L. 1996. "St. Mary's Wins McGaw Prize." *AHA News* 32 (28): 4.

McKell, D. 1994. "Primary Care Tough Issues." National Symposium on Primary Care Networks, New Orleans, January 13.

Melville, B. 1993. "Ambulatory Care Site a Vital Strategic Decision." *Health Care Competition Week* 10 (17): 1–4.

Menkin, H. L. 1994. "Physician/Managed Care Impact Analysis." Menkin Strategies/Health Forecasting Group (unpublished). April.

Pulley, M. 1994. "Mullikin and Hill Physicians in Talks About Statewide System." *Integrated Healthcare Report* (March): 15–16.

Rudd, T. 1994. "PruCare Recruits 75 PCPs in '93, Plans on 100 This Year." *Health Care Competition Week* 11 (7): 4–5.

Sardinha, C. 1995. "Capitation Offers Biggest Growth Market for Medicaid HMOs, as States Forge Ahead with New Waivers." Special Report. *Managed Care Outlook* 8 (3): 1–4.

Schultz, D. V. 1994. "The Importance of Primary Care for an Integrated Healthcare Provider." National Symposium on Primary Care Networks, New Orleans, January 13.

Shinkman, R. 1995. "The Ascent of UniHealth." *California Medicine* 6 (11): 14–15.

Southwick, K. 1994. "Putting the Pieces in Place for Regional Integration." *Strategies for Healthcare Excellence* 7 (1): 1–7.

Wagner, L. 1996 "Patient Competition, Improved Negotiating Power Drives Healthcare Organizations to Develop PCNs." *Integrated Care and Capitation* 1 (9): 1–2.

CHAPTER 7

Independent Physician Organizations: Doctor-Owned Medical Networks Put Physicians in Control of Managed Care

The next five to eight years will be messy, as managed care penetration alters the power structure for everyone, including specialists and primary care physicans.... The physician organizations that will lose will include the inefficient, the clinically ineffective—or too slow to change—and those lacking leverage in the bidding process.

Doug McKell, President, Physician Strategies 2000 (1993, 3)

PHYSICIANS SHOULD take note that the coming of managed care, health reform, and capitation offers them a one-time opportunity to regain clinical autonomy and economic control. This is their chance to relegate to the past the third-party review companies telling them what they can or cannot do with patients, the laborious appeals for treatment authorization, and the retroactive denials of payment for provided services. It is possible for doctors and their patients to make all the decisions.

The means to this end is the independent physician organization (IPO). IPOs are doctor-owned, business-managed medical networks. Through them, physicians can position themselves to be partners sought after by HMOs, insurers, health systems, and hospitals. To be successful, an IPO must have the following characteristics:

- shared business vision;
- physician commitment and loyalty;
- leadership delegated to a small corporate-style board;
- decentralized network of physician providers;
- appropriate mix of primary care and specialty physicians;
- savvy business organization for contracting;
- practice management capability;
- retained earnings to capitalize expansion;
- information system and research capacity;
- agreement on treatment standards and practice guidelines;
- willingness to discipline on economic and quality grounds;
- shared risk management and insurance expense;
- preference for capitation and HMO approaches;
- clinical discipline to practice cost-efficient care;
- equitable compensation plan with incentives;
- well-chosen partnerships with HMOs or insurers; and
- regionally distributed network of quality hospitals.

More than $5 billion of Wall Street capital is fueling development of very large physician groups. Some, like MedPartners/Mullikin of Birmingham, Alabama, and PhyCor of Nashville, Tennessee, include thousands of physicians and operate in more than a dozen states. These companies have a special appeal for doctors. "It's the money!" exclaims Lance Piccolo, chairman and CEO of Caremark (Ponton 1996, 5). The money represents not just capital, but the ability to make groups better managed and more profitable, through information systems, business management, and contracting strategies. Caremark believes that its information system is worth $5 million in increased profitability for a large medical group.

DOCTORS WANT A BIGGER SHARE OF THE HEALTHCARE PIE

Physicians are seeking a bigger slice of the national health spending "pie" (see Fig. 7.1). National health expenditures reached $1 trillion in 1994, according to the U.S. Commerce Department (Kostreski 1994). The same year, physician spending climbed 11.2 percent. Doctors make up 18 percent of the healthcare economy, less than half the hospital share of 39 percent. But that is changing as doctors take control of HMO capitation contracts, increasing ambulatory

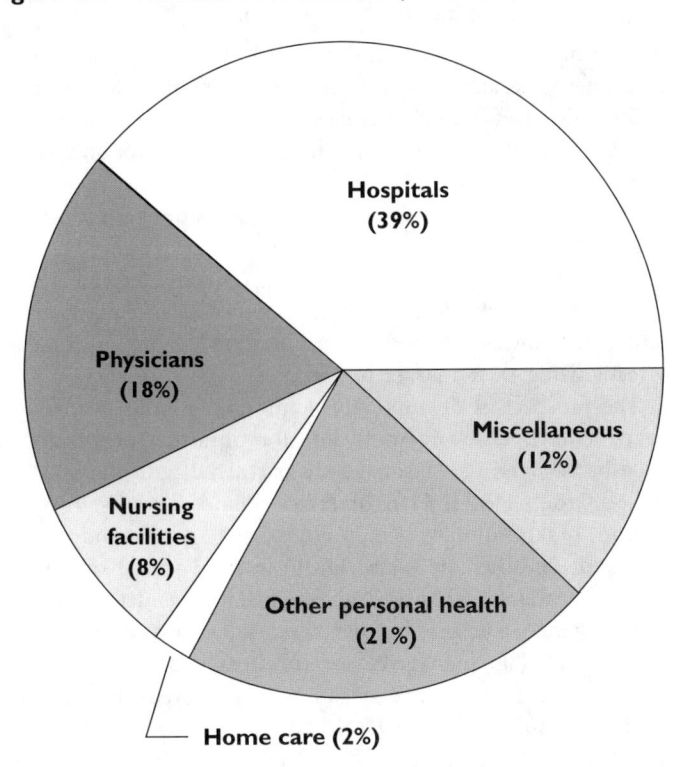

Figure 7.1 Healthcare Pie Reaches $1 Trillion

- Hospitals (39%)
- Physicians (18%)
- Nursing facilities (8%)
- Home care (2%)
- Other personal health (21%)
- Miscellaneous (12%)

Source: U.S. Commerce Department, "U.S. Industrial Outlook 1994," adapted from AHA News, *January 3, 1994.*

care while making substantial reductions in hospital admissions and lengths of stay.

For physicians to get their fair share of the healthcare economy, they must develop strong medical groups and business strategies. Doug McKell, president of Physician Strategies 2000 in Franklin, Ohio, recommends strong medicine for physicians facing managed care markets: "Providers must be more than organized; they must belong to contracting groups that possess the financial strength and management expertise to assure primary care access across multiple delivery sites, provide objective measures of patient satisfaction and clinical outcomes, and prove the effectiveness of treatments" (McKell 1993, 4).

DOCTORS MANAGING DOCTORS

The future of independent physician organizations will be built on a new basis: Doctors will manage doctors. Physicians will control the cost and content of medical care. These physician-owned organizations will aggressively seek capitation and manage the costs of care with a commitment to quality. Doctor-initiated medical networks and groups are demonstrating they can overcome the limitations of capital, management experience, information systems, practice standards, and the traditional autonomy of the doctor-patient relationship.

From coast to coast, doctor-owned organizations are constructing their own future. Boston-based Lahey Clinic, for example, struck long-term affiliations with Massachusetts General Hospital and the Harvard Community Health Plan. Strong medical organizations are naming their own price and getting preferred treatment. Doctors are recognizing their market power.

The prospect of doctors contracting for millions of managed care patients is a strong motivator for physician organizations. Seattle-based Virginia Mason Clinic partnered with the 500,000-enrollee Group Health Plan of Puget Sound. These staff-model nonprofit organizations—one an established hospital and medical group and the other the oldest HMO in the Pacific Northwest—developed a strategic alliance. Both retained independent ownership and governance structures but partnered to create a regional health plan with 420,000 managed care enrollees and three hospitals. Creating a medical alliance began with a shared culture. Both Virginia Mason and Group Health operated from a staff model. They spoke the same language, shared a vision of clinical excellence, and believed they would compete on quality. The two organizations established the Institute for Healthcare Excellence, through which they jointly developed practice guidelines and new insurance products. The next step may be clinical integration and consolidation.

THE THREAT AND REALITY OF MANAGED CARE

Physician paranoia about managed care is well grounded, after years of reduced payments and hassling with HMOs and insurers over treatment authorizations. The plans demand steep discounts and intrude deeply into the physician-patient relationship with prior authorization and third-party review. Doctors are often overmatched by insurers and HMOs, who contract with thousands of clinicians, usually at substantial reductions in physician charges. Unorganized solo physicians and small groups often find themselves at the mercy of managed care plans, as the doctors sign virtually every contract that comes through the mail slot, not knowing which plan will really deliver patients.

Physician involvement with HMOs is almost unavoidable in today's marketplace. Fifty percent of doctors have signed one HMO agreement, another 25 percent are signed up with two managed care plans, and an enterprising 13 percent are enrolled with four or more HMOs (SMG Marketing 1993). The specialty with the highest percentage of managed care contracts is, surprisingly, not general or family practice, with 63 percent. The categories with the most HMO contracts—tied at 80 percent—are surgical subspecialties and obstetrics/gynecology (see Table 7.1).

WILL PHYSICIAN ORGANIZATIONS SEEK HMO LICENSES?

As physicians organize into networks and large multispecialty groups, many will eliminate the middleman and develop their own HMOs. The rationale is easy enough to understand: Doctors are tired of being the bottom of the food chain. More and more, they are demanding to take on some or all of the insurance risk, and enjoy any financial gains from cost cutting. Large multispecialty clinics are already moving to establish their own HMOs. Seattle-based Virginia Mason's HMO has an enrollment of 40,000. The Fallon Clinic

Table 7.1 HMO Contracts and Revenue, by Clinical Specialty

Specialty	Percentage with HMO Contracts	Percentage of Revenue from HMOs
Surgical subspecialties	80	29
Obstetrics/gynecology	80	43
Internal medicine subspecialties	79	29
General surgery	77	30
Pediatrics	76	41
Radiology	72	28
General internal medicine	70	29
Anesthesiology	65	33
Pathology	65	28
General/family practice	63	35
Psychiatry	51	27
Emergency medicine	35	22
Other	61	35
All Physicians	70	32

Source: Adapted from American Medical Association. 1993. Socioeconomic Characteristics of Medical Practice. Chicago: The Association.

in Worcester, Massachusetts, Wisconsin's Marshfield Clinic, and Pennsylvania-based Geisinger Clinic have built HMOs with more than 100,000 enrollees. The American Medical Association estimates there are 3,000 physician networks. Some of the most aggressive, like Partners Community Healthcare of Boston, Massachusetts, are dropping hospital representation from their boards to become truly physician-dominated organizations. The Partners group has taken on a capitation contract from Tufts Associated Health Plans for a Medicare HMO, breaking out of its vendor status with local HMOs.

Large and successful independent physician organizations will certainly consider whether to build or buy their own HMOs. MedPartners/Mullikin, a primary care–based physician group with 1.1 million covered lives in southern California, acquired an HMO license but planned to use it only for "wholesale" global capitation contracts with HMOs. Mullikin was obviously anxious about sending "the wrong signal" to their HMO customers (Nodell 1994). Mullikin had 22 HMO agreements. Other physician groups may come to the same approach: Build HMO partnerships to get better reimbursement and avoid being punished by HMOs who would resent the doctor-owned HMO competition.

Another California medical organization, the Bay Shores Medical Group of Torrance, established a 3,000-member HMO to serve the small-employer market. Bay Shores then merged with Health Care Partners, another physician network, and the merged organization serves more than 225,000 enrollees. Physician-sponsored HMOs are a minitrend, but probably not a major strategy for physician organizations, believes Jim Hillman, executive director of United Medical Group, a trade association of large managed care medical organizations (Nodell 1994).

Vertical integration will encourage doctor networks into strategic alliances with hospitals and health systems. There have been expensive failures of doctor-owned HMOs that could not control costs, including Bay State in Massachusetts and the Health Plan of Greater San Diego. Some experts feel it would be "suicide" for doctor networks to compete with HMOs. Andrew Larkowich of Kenneth Laventhal & Co. cautions, "Even if they could get a license, there is just too much financial risk" (Nodell 1994, 12).

GROUP PRACTICES WITHOUT WALLS

With most physicians still in solo practice or two-doctor partnerships, medicine needs transitional strategies to organize for managed care. The group practice without walls (GPWW) is a single professional corporation that merges the practices of single practitioners and small groups but keeps them in their private offices while the group contracts on their mutual behalf.

The Baltimore Medical Group is such a practice, developed in an "emerging" managed care marketplace by anticipating that buyers (employers and government) wanted integrated delivery *systems* of doctors with unassailably low cost, broad geographic coverage, and vertical integration (Kimmel 1994). Baltimore physicians faced a rapidly changing market. More than 1 million Baltimore-area residents were enrolled in managed care (HMO or PPO) plans, with 40 percent in Medicare HMOs. Surrounded by deep-pocketed competitors like Johns Hopkins, the Baltimore Medical Group was launched by a handful of primary care physicians. They targeted 15 potential physician partners who met the criteria of appropriate utilization patterns, patient orientation, flexibility, and potential agreement with group principles. The result was that 10 of the 15 doctors joined the new medical group.

The survival question for these loosely structured groups is whether they can function cost-effectively and with discipline. Early experiments with group practices without walls suffered from high overhead costs and a cumbersome one-doctor-one-vote governance structure. The Baltimore Medical Group is more savvy, defining itself as a "Multilocation true group practice structured to create a culture in which previously independent physicians can evolve in a unified team approach. Essential to this is the philosophical view that a GPWW is an evolutionary step towards an integrated delivery system" (Kimmel 1994).

Dr. Alan Kimmel calls the group-practice-without-walls concept a "half-way house for fully integrated groups." He credits the Baltimore Medical Group's success to the principles of:

- provision of high quality primary care services;
- creation of their own network of specialty physicians that the group personally knew would provide quality;
- formation of a true group practice with a common information and billing system;
- controlling costs through internal utilization review and quality assurance;
- regional growth of a multisite network, with physicians clustered around multiple hospitals;
- encouraging close working relations between doctors and hospitals; and

- moving toward the ultimate development of an integrated delivery system. (Kimmel 1994)

The Baltimore Medical Group is a for-profit group entity. Its members must agree to abide by internal standards of utilization review (UR) and quality assurance (QA). Primary care physicians are employed by the group and may purchase equity, but specialists are limited in their ability to purchase equity. Specialty physicians may be employed or under contract and must assent to the group's UR/QA system. Governance is by physicians, with a voting board made up entirely of doctors. After startup with a "borrowed" set of bylaws and a line of credit from a local hospital, the Baltimore Medical Group restructured into a second-generation GPWW. Today, it is expanding into a regional delivery network of primary care group practices dispersed across the greater Baltimore area.

THE MINNESOTA PLAN FOR CLINICS WITHOUT WALLS

Minnesota may be the most competitive healthcare market in the nation, with a high level of managed care penetration and strong employer coalitions. Rapid integration among providers and the downsizing of physician networks there are spurring independent physicians to band together in new arrangements. Recent mergers between the Twin Cities HMOs with provider organizations further threaten the status of solo physicians and small medical groups. Minnesota hospitals are aggressively purchasing physician practices and groups. The Fairview Health System in Minneapolis created a closed-panel PHO in 1993 that demanded exclusivity from its physicians. Fairview doctors could not join the PHO if they also belonged to a similar organization sponsored by the rival HealthSpan system.

To help Minnesota physicians organize for health reform and managed care, the largest medical societies in the state have taken the lead in defining principles for organizing clinics without walls (Minnesota Medical Association 1993). Working jointly, the Minnesota Medical Association, Hennepin County Medical Society, and Ramsey County Medical Society developed a framework for independent physician organizations that could participate in physician-hospital organizations, integrated service networks, and other managed care arrangements.

The suggested components of the Minnesota model for a clinic without walls (CWW) include:

Corporate structure. A variety of corporate or partnership structures are possible in this model, but the recommended model is a for-profit corporation to provide the structure through which business ventures can be undertaken, including managed care contracting.

Financing and capital. Capitalization of the clinic can come from issuing stock to underwrite startup costs, while ongoing activities are funded through fees for services as well as by a management fee, such as a percentage of revenues, for managed care contracts.

Services. The for-profit corporation supports the affiliated physician practices with services such as:

- group marketing;
- third-party contract negotiations;
- cross-coverage arrangements;
- regulatory compliance;
- utilization review and quality assurance;
- data gathering and analysis, and management information system;
- strategic planning;
- practice management;
- personnel management systems; and
- central purchasing.

Contracting. An essential element of the CWW concept is economic risk sharing. The clinic must demonstrate a substantial degree of risk sharing among the physicians to avoid antitrust issues.

Network. A decentralized network of affiliated physician practices is intended to meet market demands for access by purchasers whose employees or enrollees live and work throughout the metropolitan area.

Practice autonomy. Physicians continue to manage their own practices. Pension and profit-sharing plans can remain intact, if structured properly. Methods for sharing overhead and income distribution within the practices are not controlled by the clinic.

Database. A management information system is essential for coordinating care and providing the linkages among physicians participating in the clinic network. All patients will be enrolled in a shared database, with appropriate safeguards for data privacy and confidentiality.

Utilization review and quality assurance. In support of managed care arrangements, the clinic will provide centralized utilization review and quality assurance programs. The care management process will verify at the time of service the accuracy and appropriateness of diagnoses and treatments.

Gatekeepers. To meet the expectations of purchasers, networks need a minimum of 60 percent primary care physicians to provide and coordinate care. Each patient will select a primary care doctor or medical group. Access to specialists is conditional upon referral from gatekeepers.

Physician base. A CWW is a multispecialty group practice with a strong primary care orientation. An estimated 187 doctors will be needed to serve 100,000 enrolled patients, including:

Primary care physicians	77
Medical specialists	39
Surgical specialists	45
Hospital-based specialists	26
Total	187

A base of several hundred physicians will be needed to generate this level of service, because few physicians will initially spend 100 percent of their time serving patients contracted through the clinic.

Credentialing. A process of physician selection and credentialing should bring together physicians who are compatible, committed to delivering cost-effective healthcare, and not averse to the risks of a complex business venture. Credentialing criteria will include geographic considerations, information on the cost and quality of services to existing patients, and the willingness of applicants to adhere to practice guidelines adopted by the clinic. In general, a clinics without walls should not "split" practices, with exceptions for physicians with special clinical skills.

The development of CWWs is still unfolding in Minnesota, but the state legislature has delayed the implementation of state health reform. Many Twin Cities physicians are hedging their bets with physician-hospital organizations. Some physicians have sought direct hospital employment to gain security. Others are joining large physician groups like Aspen, which affiliated with Minnesota Blue Cross, or the Park Nicollete Clinic, which merged with Methodist Hospital. In the highly evolved Twin Cities marketplace, the CWW concept may be too little, too late, as more integrated HMO organizations like HealthPartners and Allina come to dominate the market.

HENRY FORD EXPANDS FROM STAFF TO NETWORK MODEL

Detroit-based Henry Ford Health System is now pursuing a variety of physician network development initiatives. Once a staff-model organization employing all its physicians, Henry Ford had to adapt its structure to accommodate rapid expansion in the past 10 years. For Henry Ford to ride the capitation wave successfully, it has had to be more flexible with arrangements for participation in its primary care network. The emphasis on a primary care network with a variety of partners is a new paradigm for the staff-model organization.

To serve its fast-growing HMO, Henry Ford needed to develop a regional delivery network. In the 1980s, the Henry Ford system grew rapidly through acquisition of community hospitals whose medical staffs were skeptical of staff-model arrangements. Henry Ford built its primary care network using community-based family practitioners and internists. Henry Ford created a training pipeline for primary care physicians through acquisition of a family practice residency program. Today, Henry Ford relies on a network of varying local arrangements with its hospitals, including management service organizations and physician-hospital organizations.

ANTITRUST MAY BE A BARRIER TO MEDICAL MEGA-MERGERS

Putting together a mega-group to dominate a medical market is tempting but carries antitrust risk. Federal guidelines, unveiled by Hillary Rodham Clinton in 1993, provide physicians with a safety zone wherein physician networks comprise less than 20 percent of the physicians in the relevant geographic market (Melville 1993a). To avoid scrutiny for price setting, physician network members must share substantial financial risk.

These federal guidelines have only aroused physician concerns about antitrust risk in building large medical groups and networks. According to antitrust attorney John Miles of the American Medical Association's Medical Staff Legal Advisor, physician mergers can draw federal antitrust scrutiny if they meet any of the following criteria:

- The acquired practice has assets or annual net sales of $100 million or more, and the acquiring practice has at least $10 million in total assets or net sales.
- The acquired practice has assets or annual net sales of $10 million, and the acquiring group has at least $100 million in assets or net revenues.
- The acquiring practice would obtain 15 percent or more of the voting securities or assets of the acquired practice or

would obtain voting securities or assets exceeding $15 million (Melville 1993a).

Medical mergers that meet any of these criteria must report the proposed transaction to the Federal Trade Commission, accompanied by a $25,000 filing fee, and the merging partners must hold off consummating the deal for 30 days. The FTC may extend that delay if it wants more information, and the parties must wait an additional 20 days after providing the requested data.

Attorney John Miles suggests there are some simple tests of potential antitrust scrutiny:

Competitor or noncompetitor. If radiologists merge with anesthesiologists, there is no antitrust problem, but an all-radiology merger might draw review if the combined group could establish a dominant market position. A merger between multispecialty groups requires more complex analysis of its effect on competition.

Services. If a merger may affect the service mix available in the community, it may draw scrutiny. The FTC may look at broadly defined services, such as cardiology, or it may consider a service as product-specific, such as diagnostic cardiac catheterization.

Geographic territory. In determining whether or not they constitute 20 percent of the market, physicians must anticipate the FTC's view of what that market is. The "relevant geographic market" will include all territory served by the merging entities. The "relevant product market" looks more specifically at market alternatives available to third-party purchasers. The more specialized the services, the larger the relevant market must be (Melville 1993a).

LOOKING FORWARD: COULD HOSPITAL ATTITUDES BE DRIVING PHYSICIANS INTO IPOs?

The formation of independent physician organizations may be a direct result of hospital actions to try to control the marketplace. More than 3,000 hospitals and health systems have established physician-hospital organizations to position themselves for managed care contracting and national health reform, according to a study by Witt/Kiefer, Ford, Handelman & Lloyd (Melville 1993b). But only 29 percent of medical group practices are involved in PHOs. The study results are a signal. Physicians are fearful and hesitant to become involved with integrated entities.

Here are some of the reasons why hospitals may be driving physicians toward independence, not integration:

- *Moving too fast.* The rush to integration is leaving many physicians out. Hospitals are moving too quickly to establish physician-hospital organizations.
- *Top-down approach.* Physician reluctance to join physician-hospital organizations may be understandable. Doctors see PHOs as being hospital-driven.
- *Alienation of specialists.* Hospitals' emphasis on primary care as the foundation of PHOs is alienating medical specialists.
- *Purchasing instead of partnering.* Hospitals purchasing physician practices are driving away doctors who might want partnership relationships. These doctors fear hospitals will acquire enough physicians to serve the managed care contracts and close the medical staff.
- *Lack of practice management expertise.* Managing physician practices is a different business than managing hospitals. Without experienced practice managers to staff their PHOs, hospitals can quickly lose credibility with physicians.

Physician reluctance to join hospital-driven integration efforts is widespread. Kiefer/Witt, a Chicago-area search firm, found that 56.9 percent of hospitals, 76.8 percent of multihospital systems, and 45.2 percent of medical group practices have an integrated delivery system or plan to have one in the next year. According to Dan Ford of Kieffer/Witt, doctors are seeing their worlds changing and they want control over their future. Ford advises hospitals to "Convey that you're in this together" (Melville 1993b, 3).

The real challenge is getting quality physicians to join any physician network. Many quality physicians already have established practices and stable incomes. With full waiting rooms of fee-for-service patients, these doctors may be understandably slow to embrace capitation (Dickinson 1994). The next three to five years will be a battle for physician commitment and involvement. Hospitals and independent physician organizations will compete to enroll doctors in their networks. Hospitals and health systems would be smart to become partners with their doctors—and the independent physician organizations—to share jointly the risks and rewards of the era of health reform.

STRATEGIES FOR PROVIDERS, HMOs, AND SUPPLIERS

Providers

The strategic question for independent physician organizations is whether they should cooperate or compete with hospitals. Both responses are likely. Hospitals, despite their deep pockets, are at a disadvantage with capitated IPOs. The doctors can choose virtually any hospital to subcontract. The leverage is with the independent physicians. But physicians risk alienating their natural ally, potentially sacrificing the leverage that united providers might have with payers in managed care contracting. The ideal solution is a true business partnership between independent physician organizations and hospitals. Together, doctors and hospitals can share capitation and risk, control the biggest cost center (hospital), and share the rewards of reduced hospital use. Hospitals can assist their IPO partners with capital, management, legal advice and consultation, information systems, and the strength of a multihospital network.

HMOs

Many HMOs will contract directly with independent physician organizations. Teaming up with the doctors gives the HMOs two-against-one leverage in contracting with hospitals, with the hospitals losing. The result will be discounted per diem payments or low capitation rates to the hospitals. Where IPOs do not exist, HMOs may subsidize their formation. But the test of the HMO-IPO relationship will be performance. IPOs must demonstrate their ability to reduce costs, achieve quality outcomes, and satisfy customers. If not, the HMOs may show no loyalty to the IPOs, switching medical groups with no advance warning or creating HMO-owned primary care networks.

Suppliers

Independent physician organizations are a new customer for suppliers. They are also a complicating factor if the IPOs are not affiliated with existing hospital systems or group purchasing organizations. Suppliers and distributors will need to identify and develop business relationships with IPOs. Even then, the IPOs may have only limited control over drugs and supply purchases. Suppliers may want to team up with distributors, closer to the provider scene, to create business relationships with IPOs.

SOURCES

American Medical Association. 1993. "Managed Care Contracting Activity and Revenues by Specialty, 1992." *Report on Physician Trends* 1 (10): 5.

Dickinson, R. A. 1994. "Jumping the Hurdles That Get in the Way of Successful Physician-Hospital Alliances." *Medical Staff Strategy Report* 3 (1): 1–2.

Kimmel, A. 1994. "Growing a Primary Care Group Practice." National Symposium on Primary Care Networks, New Orleans, January 13.

Kostreski, F. 1994. "Health Care Spending Will Top $1 Trillion in 1994: Report." *AHA News* (30) 1: 1.

McKell, D. C. 1993. "Managed Care is Rewriting Market Rules for Hospitals and Physicians." *Report on Physician Trends* 1 (10): 3–4.

Melville, B. 1993a. "Docs Say New Antitrust Guidelines Don't Cover Enough of Their Concerns." *Health Care Competition Week* 10 (20): 4–5.

———. 1993b. "Integrated Delivery Has Already Started, But Doctors Have Some Reservations." *Health Care Competition Week* 10 (20): 3.

Minnesota Medical Association. 1993. "Clinic Without Walls Concept." *Minnesota Medicine* (June): 55.

Nodell, B. 1994. "Will Physician Groups Seek HMO Licenses?" *Northern California Medicine* 5 (2): 12.

Ponton, K. T. 1996. "How Capital Markets View Your Strategies." *Integrated Healthcare Report* 5 (5): 1–6.

SMG Marketing. 1993. "More Physicians Have Joined Multiple HMO Plans." *Report on Physician Trends* 1 (10): 4.

CHAPTER 8

Statewide Networks: Providers Organize Mega-Systems to Dominate State Markets

I've had a host of calls from payers that wanted to work out a proactive arrangement. They all start out the conversation with, "If we could both reduce our administrative costs and work together, then this [statewide network] could be a good thing."

Quentin Cook, President, California Health Network (Droste 1994a)

THE NEXT wave of healthcare restructuring will be the creation of statewide networks of hospitals, physicians, and health plans. Regional networks are not big enough to negotiate at the statewide level, where contracts may cover 1 million enrollees, and more. The biggest market targets from now until the end of the century will be mega-deals cut on a statewide basis, including:

- employer coalitions of health plans protected by the Employee Retirement Income Security Act of 1974;
- state Medicaid programs with over 30 million eligibles;
- major statewide employers, such as state governments and utilities;
- health plans and HMOs with exclusive provider agreements; and
- state-sponsored health reform, as in Oregon and Tennessee.

Providers and health plans need more "supplier's clout" with big buyers, like the California Public Employees Retirement System, which buys healthcare for 950,000 covered lives. With its purchasing power, CalPERS slashed 1993 health spending to 1.5 percent inflation, won a 2.5 percent price cut from 22 HMOs in 1994, then reduced premiums further in 1995 (Anders 1995). Even Kaiser, which covers 40 percent of CalPERS enrollees, was forced to accept a 7.5 percent rate rollback. In 1996, some of California's largest HMOs resisted pressure from CalPERS for additional price cuts. This may open the door for CalPERS to contract directly with California providers who are organizing two statewide networks and to search for HMOs and large employers who may get into statewide contracting in the future.

ECONOMIC RATIONALE FOR A STATEWIDE NETWORK

Creating statewide networks is likely to be a highly political and costly process. Why will successful regional networks come together to create statewide organizations? Analyst Adrian Zytkoskee of Adventist Health System/West identifies the strategic advantages of the statewide IDS (Droste 1994a):

Statewide contracting. The network allows sponsoring systems to manage risk on a local, regional, and, ultimately, state level. It also offers an advantage if the government moves to establish statewide health alliances under healthcare reform.

Strengthening local and regional systems. The statewide network greatly enhances providers' ability to build strong local and regional organizations.

Synergy. Statewide networks are opportunities for participants to bring different strengths and system components to the table. Regional systems that enter into partnerships benefit from each other's investments in managed care infrastructure, such as HMOs, PPOs, and medical foundations.

Information systems. Sophisticated state-level buyers demand performance accountability. That requires data compatibility across a statewide network of providers and health plans. Information systems of this scope can cost $50 million to $100 million and more. System sharing of capital costs, software, and expertise leverages all parties' information system investments.

AT-RISK PROVIDER NETWORKS COMPETE WITH HMOs

Through global capitation, hospitals and physicians compete with insurers and HMOs on a statewide basis. Physician-hospital organizations target the intermediaries—the insurers and HMOs—by developing integrated provider networks that can contract to provide all needed health services. The goal is to control enrollees, channel patients to their own provider network, and keep more of the profits that HMOs and insurers take off the top of the health benefit premium.

In direct contracting, providers bear more risk and get more of the premium dollar, up to 92 percent (Kertesz and Wojcik 1994). Cutting administrative costs—now estimated at 23 percent of all U.S. healthcare spending—is the fastest way to improve profitability and become more price-competitive.

The rationale of purchasers—HMOs, insurance plans, and self-insured employers—for capitating providers is simple: the control of health costs. Once providers accept a global capitation premium, they assume all financial risk. The rewards for capitated risk taking can be substantial. Many HMOs take 15 to 25 percent of the premium for administrative expenses and profits, although most are closer to the national average for HMO administrative costs of 12.3 percent, with 5.2 percent in operating margin for profitability (Hamer 1994).

Risk-bearing PHOs are now being criticized as "unlicensed insurance companies." A few states have established minimum capitalization requirements for PHOs (Kertesz and Wojcik 1994). Minnesota requires community-based integrated service networks that provide prepaid services for 50,000 or fewer enrollees to maintain a minimum net worth of at least $1 million. The state of Washington requires PHOs to have at least $1.5 million in capital.

To be successful, networks must demonstrate their quality and cost-effectiveness. The Joint Commission on Accreditation of Healthcare Organizations (JCAHO) is gearing up to certify integrated networks of hospitals and physicians in the future (Burda 1994a). Recognizing the widening trend among hospitals for affiliation, JCAHO's board approved a set of network accreditation standards in 1994. Network-level accreditation could streamline the process hospitals must endure in coping with the standards.

FIVE MODELS FOR STATEWIDE NETWORKS

Model 1. Nonprofit Hospital Network

About 85 percent of the nation's 5,500 community hospitals are nonprofits. Many are part of an estimated 250 integrated delivery systems and 500 network affiliations (Kertesz and Wojcik 1994). They are following the lead of pioneering integrated systems like

Sharp HealthCare in San Diego. Sharp's six hospitals and more than 600 physicians contract with 45 HMOs and insurers for 280,000 covered lives. Sharp has been a leading partner in developing the California Health Network (CHN), together with Sutter Health of Sacramento, California Healthcare System in the San Francisco Bay Area, and Adventist/West and Loma Linda University in Los Angeles. The four systems represent 1.2 million covered lives, and 15,000 affiliated physicians. Robert Montgomery, CEO of the Alta Bates Health System in Berkeley, describes CHN as a "managed care contracting network. . . . We basically want to sell the way the buyer wants to buy" (Droste 1994a).

In Kentucky, two of the state's largest nonprofit health systems formed UNIVA, a strategic alliance in September 1994 (Burda 1994b). Though the partnership was later dissolved, the strategic partnership between Baptist Healthcare System and Alliant Health System would have created a powerful nonprofit competitor to Columbia/HCA.

Chicago's healthcare networks are expanding to the fringes of the metropolitan area in deals that may create the hubs of future statewide networks (Japsen 1994). Northwestern Health Care Network added 400-bed Northwest Community Hospital in Arlington Heights, as network CEO Bruce Spivey, M.D., predicted the ultimate network size at 12 or more facilities. The network brings Medicare and Medicaid managed care products to market. Another Chicago-based network is shaping up with the merger of Lutheran General HealthSystem of Park Ridge and EHS Health Care of Oak Brook, who combined their $1.2 billion in revenues to create Advocate Health Care, a provider network able to serve the entire Chicago region. The new organization is aggressively pursuing joint managed care strategies. The physician-hospital organization of Lutheran General has experience with almost all risks, except for out-of-area emergencies and transplants. Lutheran purchases its own reinsurance and conducts in-house quality assurance and utilization management. The Advocate regional system will be a key element in a future statewide nonprofit network.

Harris Methodist of Fort Worth, Texas, is in the midst of a 10-year strategic plan to become a statewide integrated delivery system by the year 2000. Harris has a business vision of its future on a statewide level, and a long-range action plan. Networking, for Harris Methodist, is more than deal-making: "Mergers are largely driven by economic issues," states Harris' managing director Stephen Mason, "but outcomes and customer satisfaction can't be overlooked in the rush to build a network" (Greene 1994). The Harris Methodist Health Plan HMO projects enrollment of 600,000 to 700,000 in the Dallas–Ft. Worth area by 1998. The eight-hospital system is actively developing partnerships with other physicians, other hospitals, and insurers to enlarge its regional organization into a statewide system.

Model 2. For-profit Hospital Chains

For-profit hospital chains are merging and expanding at a dizzying pace. In 1994, at the height of the wave of mergers and acquisitions, there were five blockbuster deals. HealthTrust acquired Epic Healthcare for $1 billion. Columbia/HCA Healthcare Corp. purchased HealthTrust. National Medical Enterprises merged with American Medical International. OrNda acquired Summit. And Community Health Systems of Houston acquired 18 hospitals from Hallmark Healthcare. Although consolidation has slowed, as the major companies digest their growth, more large-scale mergers are likely.

Columbia/HCA eclipsed the competition with its blockbuster merger with HealthTrust. The merged company owns approximately 350 hospitals on a national basis. More important, its facilities are concentrated in the South and West, giving Columbia/HCA the potential to create statewide networks in nine states, including Texas, Florida, Kentucky, Louisiana, Georgia, Alabama, Tennessee, South Carolina, and Virginia. In Florida, Columbia/HCA owns approximately 60 facilities, so the company can boast that 90 percent of Florida's residents are within a 20-minute drive of a Columbia facility (Pogue 1995). The merger with Health Trust gave Columbia a substantial boost in new markets. For example, HealthTrust's six hospitals in Utah give Columbia a for-profit alternative to nonprofit InterMountain Health Care, which owns 19 of Utah's 41 acute facilities (Rudd 1994).

The aggressive stance of Columbia/HCA is inspiring nonprofit hospitals and systems to create statewide networks of their own. Douglas Hough of Herman Smith in Detroit observes that Columbia/HCA and the large for-profit chains "have the effect of shaking up other providers and systems—in some cases propelling them to consolidate and affiliate and create new alliances" (Lumsden and Hagland 1994).

Richard Scott, CEO of Columbia/HCA, articulates his national strategy to create regional and statewide provider networks:

- Purchase hospitals, surgicenters, and other providers in a market to create a seamless, integrated system.
- Add other providers through joint ventures or management contracts to fill out the network.

- Centralize administration of all provider entities, consolidate purchasing, negotiate to reduce outside administrative expenses, and consolidate ancillary services such as laboratory and laundry.
- Compete on price as an integrated system within each market with all buyers of healthcare.
- Offer physicians an opportunity to become equity partners in Columbia/HCA operations in their local markets.
- Give management performance incentives, with equity opportunities for senior managers.
- Where there is too much capacity, buy up competitors and shut them down. (Flower 1995)

For-profit systems may affiliate with nonprofits in developing statewide networks. Columbia/HCA's partnership with Tulane University in New Orleans and the Medical University of South Carolina in Charleston created a hub-and-spoke model that became the largest statewide network across Louisiana and created a solid base for expansion in South Carolina. In another nonprofit/for-profit alliance, Portland-based Brim, a for-profit operator of rural hospitals that manages 62 hospitals and owns 5 acute facilities, entered into partnership with SSM Health Care System of St. Louis, a Catholic health system with 17 facilities. Their goal was to develop community health networks that would align Brim's rural hospitals with SSM's urban medical centers.

Model 3. Provider-Payer Partnerships

Insurance plans and HMOs are creating statewide networks through strategic alliances with hospital systems. In Cleveland, Blue Cross and Blue Shield of Ohio linked with Meridia Health System, the largest private hospital group in the region (Jaklevic 1994). Blue Cross holds a majority interest in a for-profit managed care venture with Meridia. The Ohio Blues have also moved toward affiliating with 474-bed St. Luke's Medical Center, and Blue Cross announced a similar venture with Riverside Hospital in Toledo. The deals are part of the Blues plan's initiative to form a statewide provider network. In August 1996, policyholders of the Ohio Blues approved a joint venture with Columbia/HCA under which Columbia would acquire many assets of Blue Cross and Blue Shield of Ohio. The venture is presently undergoing regulatory review.

Many payers are now looking for statewide delivery systems for future partnerships. In Dallas, the Kaiser Permanente Health Plan recently announced an exclusive arrangement with Columbia/HCA to provide inpatient care to its 125,000 enrollees in the Dallas metropolitan area. With almost 50 hospitals in Texas, Columbia/HCA/HealthTrust could provide a statewide hospital network for future Kaiser expansion beyond its existing markets in Dallas and San Antonio.

HMOs and insurers hold a major market advantage over provider-sponsored networks. HMOs and insurers hold the enrollees, and they are beginning to adapt to PHO competition. Cigna, Aetna, and Prudential are acquiring physicians and establishing insurer-owned primary care networks. In New Jersey, Blue Cross/Blue Shield and PHP Healthcare are jointly developing a statewide primary care network (Pulley 1994). The Blues are contracting with PHP to design, build, and manage 10 primary care family health centers staffed by its own physicians. The Blues already own two primary health centers. The strategy follows creation of HMO Blue in 1993, as the Blues shift their 2 million enrollees from indemnity to managed care. The Blues' strategy to compete—not affiliate—with providers is consistent with its dropping of one-third of New Jersey's 85 hospitals and two-thirds of the state's physicians when it created HMO Blue.

Model 4. Physician-Driven Networks

Physician-driven networks may have a sustainable competitive advantage: physician loyalty. Speaking candidly, Dr. Paul Wasserstein, a board member of California Health System, stated, "Physicians can't trust anyone but other physicians" (Droste 1994b). Southern California's Friendly Hills HealthCare Network manages more than 100,000 covered lives under global capitation contracts with 27 HMOs and insurance companies. The physician group accepts all hospital and medical services risk but does not do marketing or administration.

In the long term, physicians will be the central cohesive element of tomorrow's healthcare (Goldsmith 1995). Physicians are pursuing a number of constructive ways to preserve some measure of control over their practice environment. The real force in developing integrated delivery systems is physician leadership. Only doctors have the skill to contain the cost of care and the ability to lower health expenditures without damaging the health system or its patients.

Doctors are taking the lead in IDS formation. The rise of managed care will favor primary care–based physician groups, believes Dr. Jacques Sokolov, chair of Coastal Physician Group (Engstrom 1995). Medical groups need to take a market-minded stance in developing the right mix of primary and specialty physicians. Sokolov recommends building a medical network around a primary care hub, then letting the primary care physicians select the specialists, as one of the best ways to create an optimum provider mix.

Market-minded specialty physicians are responding to the threats and opportunities of managed care by developing statewide networks. The specialists are positioning to contract for patients on a specialty carveout basis, organizing loose-knit networks and independent practice associations, and merging practices (Jaklevic 1994b). Dallas-based Texas Oncology has organized 127 physicians and 45 locations statewide in a cancer diagnostic and treatment network. Nine full-service oncology service centers offer a full range of modalities. The next step will be expansion into four other states. The physician-driven oncology network is now thinking about creating a national company and has attracted venture capital support.

Southern California's Friendly Hills HealthCare Network made headlines in 1993 when it became the first physician-driven integrated delivery system to have its nonprofit tax status approved by the Internal Revenue Service (Droste 1994c). Less than two years later, Friendly Hills reversed its course, selling its assets to for-profit Caremark International, a nationwide physician management corporation, which merged with MedPartners of Birmingham, Alabama. As participants in a Wall Street–backed for-profit company, Friendly Hills' physicians will be offered profit-sharing and the potential opportunity to participate in the "upside growth" of MedPartners/Caremark's stock.

Model 5. Staff-Model HMOs

The largest staff-model HMO in America is the Kaiser Permanente Health Plan, with 6.6 million enrollees in 12 regions. Kaiser is the model of an integrated delivery system, combining hospital, medical, insurance, and marketing services in a single organization. Kaiser generally employs its own physicians, through the Kaiser Permanente Medical Group, and owns many of its hospitals. Despite its 50-year history, Kaiser faces stiff competition from other network-model HMOs that do not have Kaiser's overhead of fully owned hospitals and employed physicians, leading Kaiser's managers to raise the possibility of outsourcing some of the needs for physicians and hospital beds. Kaiser has a well-developed statewide system in metropolitan areas of California, divided administratively into northern and southern California regions.

Other staff-model HMOs are poised for statewide expansion, taking advantage of their physician base, capital, and management systems. Detroit's Henry Ford Health Systems is creating a statewide health plan in partnership with Blue Cross of Michigan and the Sisters of Mercy in Farmington Hills. Large staff-model clinics could be the organizers of statewide networks in a number of states, including the Mayo Clinic in Minnesota, Geisinger Clinic in Pennsylvania, and Ochsner Clinic in Louisiana.

FINDING STATEWIDE PARTNERS: CRITERIA FOR NETWORKING

The creation of statewide networks is an exercise in strategy and diplomacy. It is assumed that many hospitals and health systems must participate in a statewide network to maintain market position and will need partnerships with other hospitals and systems to develop a comprehensive, strategically located continuum of care. These are among the criteria that are important in the selection of partners:

Shared values. As a value-driven system, network organizers will place much importance on a shared vision and shared values. Some hospitals and systems will have a religious affiliation, and their partners must value and respect their traditions. Religious-sponsored hospitals will want to maintain religious symbols, chaplaincy services, and other important religious connections. All partners must share a commitment to such values as community service, patient-centered care, and a holistic orientation.

Strategic locations. An important strategic and marketing strength for statewide networks will be the locations of regional hub hospitals. Potential partners will be sought that own or manage regional medical centers in key markets around the state to fill out a comprehensive statewide network. These facilities will be the central to regional hospital-physician networks.

Physician partnership. A statewide network must be constructed with a strong physician organization. Potential hospital or health system partners should bring medical organizations with managed care experience, willing to contract in a concerted statewide strategy and willing to assume risk and capitation.

HMO license or managed care plan. Ideally, hospital or health system partners will bring to the network an HMO license or equity interests in HMOs or other managed care products (e.g., PPO or third-party administrator). To compete in a managed care marketplace, network partners must be willing to commit significant capital on a multi-year basis to managed care strategies, including an HMO license, purchasing smaller regional health plans such as PPOs, and hiring top-quality HMO management.

Numbers of hospitals. Many statewide networks will initially be constructed by alliances between established health systems. Other hospital or health system partners will be needed to fill in the map for a decentralized delivery system across the state, including every subregion. This assumes that major purchasers and insurers will want a statewide system with well-distributed hospitals. This will also position the regional networks for contracting with local employers and purchaser coalitions.

Tertiary partner. Every statewide network will need a partner to be the tertiary hub of the statewide IDS. The tertiary partner should be a recognized statewide leader in specialty services (e.g., cardiology, trauma, orthopedics, neurology, oncology). Ideally, the tertiary partner will also bring a transportation network such as a helicopter or fixed-wing air ambulance service.

Commitment to quality. All network partners must demonstrate dedication to quality, with Total Quality Management/Continuous Quality Improvement programs and a high level of management, board, and medical staff commitment to quality. Facilities in the partnership must be willing to share data and participate in benchmarking programs.

Capital. IDS partners should be willing to commit significant capital to developing a statewide network. A five-year budget for IDS development may be $50 million to $100 million for physician networks, information systems, and managed care strategies.

Low-cost position. To be competitive, hospitals and health systems entering a statewide network must be committed to achieving a low-cost market position. That means a willingness to cut costs and, if necessary, close services or facilities to make the total network clinically efficient.

Information system. All parties will share an integrated information network. Network partners must be willing to work rapidly to achieve information system compatibility. Costs of achieving information integration are essential investments.

BUILDING NETWORKS THROUGH MERGERS AND ACQUISITIONS

Some statewide networks will be built the old-fashioned way—through mergers and acquisitions. The pace of deal-making is picking up rapidly. In response to the moves by Columbia/HCA, Tenet, and OrNda to form mega-companies in 1994, the number of mergers and acquisitions among acute hospitals rose. Small hospitals and struggling urban facilities are going for as little as

$2 million to $3 million, while suburban facilities in better locations are fetching prices of $50 million to $60 million.

Most hospitals are being purchased by other hospitals or multihospital systems, as nonprofit and proprietary systems fill in their networks. Physician groups and HMOs are new players in the network game. Boston's Lahey Clinic, for example, paid $4 million for the Symmes Hospital in suburban Arlington, Massachusetts. In southern California, Pacific Physician Services, a publicly traded physician group practice, purchased two hospitals from National Medical Enterprises and is reselling one facility to Vencor, the Louisville-based chain of intensive-care facilities.

IS ANTITRUST A PROBLEM FOR STATEWIDE NETWORKS?

Antitrust barriers for mergers and acquisitions may be easing. In response to demands by the American Hospital Association for antitrust relief, the Federal Trade Commission and the Justice Department released revised antitrust guidelines for the health field in 1994, which expanded and clarified six "safety zones" for provider consolidation (Burda 1994a). Although legal experts are cautious about the practical effect of the new guidelines, they do expand areas for physician collaboration, up to 30 percent of a market. Additional antitrust protection for provider-sponsored networks was part of the Republican budget-balancing initiative, vetoed by President Clinton. The American Hospital Association continues to push for an antitrust shield that would allow greater provider consolidation, especially in small-hospital markets.

It is not clear yet whether networks—which, as joint ventures, involve no merger of assets—will get a different treatment from the Justice Department or the FTC. The federal agencies have not responded to the American Hospital Association's request for more clarification on the formation of multiprovider networks. Antitrust attorneys generally believe that loosely constructed networks do not present as much of an anticompetitive issue as asset-merged systems. But networks are likely to form even in the absence of definitive federal policy, with sponsors seeking federal clarification from the FTC and Justice Department and proceeding unless definitively blocked.

EMPLOYER COALITIONS COULD EXPAND STATEWIDE NETWORKS

Employers are fueling demand for statewide networks. Regional employer purchasing coalitions will emerge as state-level buyers in the next few years. In San Francisco, executives of the Pacific Business Group on Health negotiate with 17 HMOs in the nine-county Bay Area. Successful contracting at the regional level should encourage other employer coalitions in California to pool their enrollees and purchasing power, probably in excess of $2 billion to $3 billion dollars on a statewide basis.

Employer-provider partnerships are reaching new levels in Minnesota's Twin Cities. Sophisticated employers have formed two major purchasing coalitions, for large and small business firms. The large-employer coalition has worked in the past with Minneapolis-based Health Partners in managing care and quality. Purchasers and providers jointly sponsored the Institute for Clinical Systems Integration, a research and development organization to develop clinical protocols and experiment with care management approaches (Reinersten 1994). HealthSystem Minnesota, created by Methodist Hospital and the Park Nicollet Medical Center, is aligned with HealthPartners, the region's largest HMO, in what may grow into a statewide integrated services network. The direct contracting initiative launched by the large-employer Buyers Health Care Action Group in 1997 could be expanded into a statewide initiative. The state of Minnesota has joined that coalition, bringing another 100,000 covered lives that could be converted to direct contracting when the state's union contracts expire.

WILL CORPORATE-PRACTICE LAWS LIMIT NETWORKS?

Corporate-practice statutes could be a barrier to integrated networks, as hospitals employ physicians in new hospital-affiliated organizations. Virtually all states have a ban on the corporate practice of medicine, either by statute or by case law. But only 13 states have taken action to enforce the ban, according to Los Angeles–based attorney Wayne J. Miller of Weissburg and Aronson. An analysis by the firm showed another 13 states that permitted hospitals to employ doctors, with the rest of the states somewhere in the middle (Hudson 1994). National health reform could address corporate-practice-of-medicine discrepancies among the states, but the political chances of enactment seem low after the failure of the Clinton health plan in 1994.

In Tennessee, healthcare institutions unsuccessfully sought to enact a statute that would protect hospital employment of physicians. In order to participate in TennCare, the state's Medicaid reform initiative, hospitals planned to hire physicians to see TennCare patients, because many independent physicians did not want TennCare patients leaving hospitals as the providers of last resort. But the legislation was strongly opposed by the Tennessee Medical Association, which feared hospital control of patients and referrals.

California has a ban on corporate practice but permits the creation of nonprofit medical foundations, which may contract for physician services. A 1974 statute was enacted to cover existing clinics, but a number of California health systems and hospitals have used it to create a third-party entity that could contract for services with a multispecialty medical clinic. In this model, the control of the medical practice is still with the medical group, but the foundation model allows the hospital to invest capital in the growth of the physician organization.

BUILD OR BUY: WHICH IS RIGHT FOR STATEWIDE NETWORKS?

Organizers of statewide integrated delivery systems face a classic business dilemma: Should they build their organizations through asset merger and acquisition, or through affiliation? The greatest advantage of system ownership is control, that is, the ability to direct resources from a centralized management perspective. Fully owned systems pool capital and revenues, integrate human resources and strategies, and share the same information system. They are guided by a single vision of the future and integrated strategic plans to achieve their goals. Governance is simple and businesslike. A CEO has clear charge of the system, and a small corporate-style board makes quick decisions.

On the other hand, "buying" affiliates through a lattice of contracts and mutual agreements produces a network in which no one owns anything. This is an organization based on trust and backed by contracts defining roles and reimbursement. Governance is a freewheeling affair with principals from each participating organization sharing in consensus—or lack of consensus—about future directions. Managing a network is like "herding cats," by aligning the interests of stakeholders and facilitating cooperative action. Every activity in a network is a project managed by a task force.

If a merged system is "tight," then a network is "loose." Of course, it is more complicated than that. Not every hospital or physician wants to be merged or acquired. Futurist Jeff Goldsmith is vocal in his critique of the "build" strategy: "The core flaw in the integrated movement in healthcare is the use of an obsolete, 19th-century, asset-based model of integration" (Goldsmith 1994).

The capital costs of traditional asset merger and acquistions can leave the system struggling with enormous debt, making price competition difficult.

When an integrated delivery system owns all its key assets, system capital is tied up in facilities, which may limit much-needed spending to develop physician organizations or managed care products. The bureaucracy needed to manage a statewide system may impede the kind of rapid responses and quick-to-market strategies that are essential in a changing marketplace.

Goldsmith's recommendation is "virtual integration"—an organization that works like a system but without the bricks-and-mortar asset base. The virtual IDS or network model is held together by (1) an operating system of agreements and protocols for managing patients, and (2) a framework of incentives that governs how physicians and hospitals are paid. The concept is simple to understand. The principal assets are information systems and capital to construct whatever is needed to engage in managed care contracting. Networks can husband their capital to invest in an HMO license, physician organizations, or managed care software (Goldsmith 1994).

WIRING THE NETWORKS

A spiderweb of electronic linkages enables statewide networks to function. The key to survival in managed care is management of financial risk (Ruffin 1995). But building the "information highway" between network partners is not easy, inexpensive, or quickly accomplished. A panel of information systems consultants and chief information officers (CIOs) identified six key issues for IDS information network development:

- facilitating the transition to integrated delivery systems;
- making clinical information systems more useful and relevant to the clinicians;
- sorting out the role of community health information networks;
- handling security, privacy, and confidentiality concerns;
- maneuvering through vendor issues: collaboration, consolidation, and competition; and
- strengthening the role of the CIO. (Bergman 1994a)

Community health information networks will form the underlying architecture for statewide delivery networks. Experts estimate that some 100 CHINs are in partial deployment or planning stages (Bergman 1994b). Few are fully operational yet because they do not have the breadth of participants or functions. CHIN vendors include Ameritech Health Connections of Chicago, Health Communications Services in Richmond, Virginia, Integrated Medical Systems of Golden, Colorado, and Health Data Exchange of Malvern, Pennsylvania.

As CHINs become operational, they will improve quality and reduce costs by facilitating the electronic interchange of clinical and financial data. CHIN network partners will include hospitals, physicians, insurers and HMOs, and other community providers. CHIN development is a political process, but all stakeholders must ultimately collaborate if the statewide network model of integrated delivery systems is to be successful.

CAN STATEWIDE NETWORKS MEET THE CHALLENGE OF RIGHTSIZING?

America has almost 500,000 surplus beds, according to a long-term forecast by the Sachs Group (Cerne and Montague 1994). Based on hospital occupancy of 67 percent and assuming HMO use rates, the study identified a surplus of 447,545 excess hospital beds. Even if the forecast were done using rates 50 percent higher than HMO experience, there would still be at least 207,000 excess beds. Eliminating the excess capacity would be the equivalent of closing almost 2,500 community hospitals, averaging 172 beds per facility.

In trendsetting southern California, managed care has reduced use rates to record lows. The average daily census in private hospitals there was 44 percent in 1995, and more than half of the region's hospitals have operated in the red. Not counting mergers, some 40 hospitals in southern California closed between 1988 and 1993. Many failed hospitals were smaller—under 150 beds—and no longer competitive or needed. Staffers at the Healthcare Association of Southern California predict that another 15 percent of the region's hospitals will close by the year 2000.

If statewide networks are to be effective, their sponsoring health systems must be able to regionalize services and consolidate facilities. Rural facilities will be especially targeted because their small bed size makes them financially vulnerable to the decline of inpatient demand. According to the American Hospital Association's Section for Small or Rural Hospitals, 550 rural facilities stopped providing acute care between 1984 and 1991. Of these, 47 percent became specialized healthcare facilities, another 27 percent converted to another health-related purpose, and 26 percent ceased all healthcare operations. Dealing with the costs of excess capacity while maintaining a viable and accessible distribution of facilities will be a major challenge for statewide IDS networks.

LOOKING FORWARD: COMMUNICATION IS MORE IMPORTANT THAN CAPITAL

The critical success factor in starting a statewide network is communication, not capitalization. Dr. Joel Sklar, of California Health System, states bluntly, "The deals that are being struck are being struck among people who understand that they need each other" (Droste 1994b). Network sponsors must share an understanding of the future market, and a vision of what will be needed to survive and succeed. When venturing into the unknown—especially where the business risks and benefits are uncharted—partners must trust one another.

Developing statewide networks will be particularly complex because of time and distance. Local conditions within the same state can vary widely. Managed care penetration may be high in one metropolitan area and low in another city elsewhere in the state. Rural hospitals will fear dominance by large urban medical centers. Physicians with full waiting rooms may feel no need to change, while other doctors with positive HMO relations are ready to charge ahead.

Stakeholders in statewide networks will bring many different points of view:

- *Hospitals* want assured revenues and adequate volume to support their facility investment.
- *Physicians* are concerned about their income and control of patient care.
- *Academic medical centers* are feeling the loss of their center-stage position and funding for teaching and research.
- *Rural hospitals* are financially fragile and fear loss of independence.
- *HMOs and insurers* see risk-taking providers as a threat to their role as intermediary.

STRATEGIES FOR POTENTIAL PARTNERS IN STATEWIDE NETWORKS

Creating state-level coalitions from these disparate partners will be an exercise in diplomacy. Here are some specific strategies to increase communication among the parties, reduce front-end dickering, and move everyone to joint decision making:

1. *Share assumptions.* Network participants must come to share a set of assumptions about the future. A one-day session with consultants and colleagues from managed care markets can confirm the group's fears that managed care is really taking over their market.
2. *Engage in high-level discussions.* Principals must be involved as early as possible, preferably CEO to CEO.
3. *Involve physicians.* Physicians must be participants from the beginning. They are highly wary about hospital control and must be treated as partners even if there are no strong physician organizations as yet in the market.
4. *Limit goals.* The action agenda for the network must be limited, without goals that are too ambitious for the network. At this early stage, the apparatus to achieve ambitious goals does not yet exist.
5. *Capitalize.* The potential partners in statewide networks must put real money on the table immediately. In small markets, $100,000 each may be enough. For large markets, startup investments of $1 million per player may be minimal.

SOURCES

Anders, G. "CalPERS Discloses Rate Cuts of 3.8% From Health Plans," *Wall Street Journal,* 16 February 1995, p. B6.

Bergman, R. 1994a. "Health Care in a Wired World." *Hospitals & Health Networks* 68 (16): 28–36.

———. 1994b. "Data Detente: Community Health Information Networks." *Hospitals & Health Networks* 68 (12): 46–50.

Burda, D. 1994a. "No Network Surveys Scheduled—JCAHO." *Modern Healthcare* 24 (30): 3, 6.

———. 1994b. "Kentucky Systems Collaborate." *Modern Healthcare* 24 (39): 20.

Cerne, R., and J. Montague. 1994. "Capacity Crisis." *Hospitals & Health Networks* 68 (19): 30–40.

Droste, T. M. 1994a. "Statewide Healthcare Network Launches in California." *Medical Staff Strategy Report* 3 (7): 1–2.

———. 1994b. "Physician-Hospital Network Boils Down to Three Words: Communicate, Communicate, Communicate." *Medical Staff Strategy Report* 3 (8): 3–6.

———. 1994c. "Integration Leader Friendly Hills Switches Models—Again." *Hospitals & Health Networks* 68 (22): 67–68.

Engstrom, P. 1995. "Medical Group Practices Need More Than Luck in the Provider-Mix Game." *Medical Network Strategy Report* 4 (2): 1–3.

Flower, J. 1995. "Rick Scott: Icon of Greed or Leader of True Health Reform?" *Healthcare Forum Journal* 38 (2): 71–78.

Goldsmith, J. C. 1994. "The Illusive Logic of Integration." *Healthcare Forum Journal* 37 (5): 26–31.

———. 1995. "Health Care's Power Brokers in the 21st Century." *Physician Executive* 21 (1): 7–9.

Greene, J. 1994. "Begin with the End Result When Building a System." *Modern Healthcare* 24 (30): 51–52.

Hamer, R. 1994. "HMO Industry Report, Part II." *InterStudy Competitive Edge* 3 (1): 1–116.

Hudson, T. 1994. "Hospitals Work Through the Corporate Practice Maze." *Hospitals & Health Networks* 68 (19): 60–62.

Jaklevic, M. 1994a. "Ohio Blues Buy Into Deal with Cleveland Provider." *Modern Healthcare* 24 (30): 36.

———. 1994b. "Staying Single: Can Single-Specialty Group Practices Survive in Managed Care Markets?" *Modern Healthcare* 24 (40): 71–80.

Japsen, B. 1994. "Chicago Network-Building Shifting to New Suburbs as Big Chains Divvy Up Spoils." *Modern Healthcare* 24 (40): 42.

Kertesz, L., and J. Wojcik. 1994. "Risky PHO's Winning Bet." *Modern Healthcare* 24 (30): 44–48.

Lumsden, K., and M. Hagland. 1994. "For-Profits: The Right Medicine for Some Markets?" *Hospitals & Health Networks* 68 (12): 34–42.

Pogue, J. 1995. "Battlefield Florida." *Integrated Healthcare Report* 4 (11): 1–8.

Pulley, M. 1994. "New Jersey Blues to Build Primary Care Network." *Integrated Healthcare Report* 3 (4): 17.

Reinersten, J. J. 1994. "Meeting Society's Root Needs." *Healthcare Forum Journal* 68 (19): 40–44.

Rudd, T. 1994. "FTC Lets Network Grow in Utah Antitrust Settlement." *Healthcare Systems Strategy Report* 11 (15): 1–2.

Ruffin, M. 1995. "Managed Care Information Needs: A Summary Perspective." *Physician Executive* 21 (1): 44–46.

CHAPTER 9

Physician-Hospital Integration: Creating New Models of Provider Partnerships

Integration is a means to an end—not an end. The goal is to lower costs, improve clinical outcomes and service quality.

Rick Norling, President and CEO, Fairview Hospital
and Health Services (1995, 50)

THE NEXT five years of physician-hospital integration will be critical. A hospital or health system can "make its market" with partnership initiatives with its physicians, or lose market share and managed care contracts to a more proactive competitor. The ultimate goal is an integrated delivery network of hospitals and physicians that can accept and manage enrolled populations under at-risk contracts. The question for the 1990s is: Will hospitals and physicians collaborate or compete in the managed care payment food chain (Coile 1994)?

The traditional medical staff must ultimately be replaced by an economic organization that unites hospitals and physicians in a long-term business and clinical partnership. Getting to integration is more complicated. Options include:

- Joint venture between the hospital and doctors.
- The hospital purchases physician practices.
- The hospital or system creates a tax-exempt foundation.

- Physician group leases, purchases, or builds a hospital.
- The hospital is the prime contractor; physicians are subcontractors.
- Physicians are the prime contractor; the hospital is the subcontractor.
- For-profit company acquires the physicians and contracts with the hospital.

Will the provider partnership be balanced? Or controlled by one side or the other? In California, where managed care is the widespread payment format, physicians appear to dominate the relationship. On the West Coast generally, medical groups hold the primary position in HMO contracts, not hospitals. On the East Coast and elsewhere, where there are few established physician group practices, hospitals have traditionally held the balance of power over physicians.

Victoria McKemy, vice president of Summit Care in Garden Grove, California, observes, "If, indeed, physician groups feel motivated to integrate, they will be looking to find, buy, lease, or somehow acquire an acute-care hospital and/or a skilled nursing hospital" (McKemy 1995).

CHOOSING AN INTEGRATION PARTNER: PHYSICIANS OR PAYERS?

Physician-hospital integration is becoming more complicated. Now there are three players: hospitals, physicians, and payers. Third-party payers, that is, HMOs and insurers, are purchasing primary care physicians to form staff-model medical groups. In this model, the third-party payer becomes the primary care provider and gatekeeper to the hospital and to specialty care referrals. The integration of HMOs and insurers with physicians drives a wedge between hospitals and their doctors, confounding providers' local partnership activities. In a variation on this theme, some publicly traded HMOs are offering stock to physician groups to increase their loyalty. PacifiCare of California is offering Class B (nonvoting) stock to provider groups to reinforce close alliances (Cochrane 1995).

Columbia/HCA is choosing to contract with payers first, then figure out its physician partners (Rudd 1995). In Houston, the nation's largest hospital chain is not acquiring physicians. Columbia/HCA believes that managed care plans will decide where patients go. The price of creating a physician network in Houston is prohibitive, so the big chain is putting its emphasis on solidifying contractual links with insurers, HMOs, and PPOs. Instead of contracting directly with physicians, the company links itself with physician groups through payer contracts.

REAL PARTNERSHIP IS SHARING THE PREMIUM DOLLAR

The true measure of successful provider partnership strategies is the development of business relationships in which physicians and hospitals share a managed care premium. In a global capitation arrangement, in which hospitals and doctors are jointly given incentives to manage all healthcare costs, such as by sharing a risk pool for hospital expenses, the reduction in hospital expenditures benefits all the providers. Hospitals and physicians are joining together to increase their market power with HMOs and insurers, hoping to use this "supplier's clout" to win better payments and terms from HMOs in managed care contracting.

A backlash from the HMOs and insurers is emerging, however. The danger in creating provider partnerships, cautions Nathan Kaufman, a managed care consultant in San Diego, is that "Most payers view PHOs . . . as 'cartels,' and thus competitors for market power" (Kaufman 1995). Payers may limit the effectiveness of PHOs by refusing to recognize these organizations and by contracting separately with primary care physicians, specialists and hospitals. Many payers view the "provider one-stop-shop network" as a competitive threat. Some large HMOs and insurers like Aetna, Prudential, and Foundation Health Plan are acquiring their own primary care networks.

To win the battle for market power, providers must make hard decisions and move aggressively to develop the keys to managed care dominance:

- single-signature and exclusive contracting authority for all hospitals and physicians;
- contracts for and control of covered lives;
- a marketwide network of primary care physicians;
- managed care infrastructure for lower per-enrollee costs;
- clinical prestige in key services, such as obstetrics or open-heart surgery;
- advantageously located facilities and market coverage; and
- cost-effective management of chronic diseases. (Kaufman 1995)

FIVE PARTNERSHIP STRATEGIES FOR PHYSICIANS AND HOSPITALS

Strategy 1. Direct Contracting and Risk-Sharing

Cutting out the intermediary—the insurer—is not for the timid. Hospitals and physicians who cooperate to do this successfully can lock-in employer or managed care plan loyalty for multi-year contracts. But failures can be costly if volumes are low, costs are high, or discounts are too deep to cover expenses. Physician partnerships are essential. The president of a California hospital-owned medical foundation, Dr. Harry Glatstein (1993), puts it bluntly: "Purchasers are buying health care from organized medical groups—not hospitals."

"Managed competition" envisions many direct contracting relationships between employer purchasing groups and physician-hospital networks. Most direct contracting arrangements involve discounts from normal billed charges for physicians and negotiated per diem reimbursement for hospitals. Some direct contracts are based on anticipated revenues or admissions, and a few use DRG-based payment schemes. Single-service contracting is growing. Among the most popular services are obstetrics and cardiac care services, for which the hospital and physician agree to accept a single fee and to share the financial risk if costs exceed the all-inclusive price. In Chicago, a partnership of Advocate Health Care partnered with doctors to offer Behavioral Health Direct, a managed care joint venture that offers employers direct contracting for behavioral health services. Former Advocate chief executive Stephen L. Ummel describes the relationship: "We have a very strong partnership between systems, hospitals, and most important between physicians. Hospitals can't effect much change in case management, utilization, and cost without a strong partnership with the practicing physicians" (Johnsson 1992).

Failure of the Clinton plan for national health reform may strongly encourage the development of direct contracting with employer purchasing groups. Southern California Edison is an early example of direct purchasing of healthcare by a large employer. Edison constructed its own network of 85 hospitals and 7,500 physicians to serve the utility's 56,000 employees, dependents, and retirees. Direct contracting had a dramatic result in managing health costs. Edison saved $100 million in five years, with healthcare expenses some 20 percent below what the company would otherwise have spent (Sokolov 1993). Edison has returned to contracting through an intermediary, utilizing Aetna as its network manager, but on favorable multi-year terms to the employer.

Direct contracting is not for all hospitals or physicians. Perhaps 5 percent to 10 percent of the largest employers have the buying power and sophistication to engage in direct provider contracting. Hospitals often lack specific data on costs and quality on which to price their bids, and hospital information systems are often inadequate to provide the detailed reporting employers will want.

Contracting with a high-visibility employer can, however, enhance the hospital's status in managed care contracting with other major employers and insurance companies.

Strategy 2. Hub-and-Spoke Managed Care

In hub-and-spoke regional delivery systems, dominant regional medical centers develop affiliations with primary care hospitals and physicians that channel patients to the hub tertiary care facility for specialized services. Community hospitals and primary care and multispecialty medical groups are the spokes. The hub-and-spoke networks that include the area's best hospitals and top-quality physicians are the providers preferred by HMOs, PPOs, and insurance companies. Ideally, a network includes a hospital- or physician-owned HMO, PPO, or both. Then it is a fully integrated healthcare system. Networks are linked by business and clinical relationships, with shared ownership and control.

Sharing financial risk in capitation contracts is critical to the network model. But a network must share patients and revenues fairly, not relegated to being feeders to the regional hub. Alliances thrive only when relationships are perceived to provide mutual value to all participants. Early on the primary value of hub-and-spoke networks is referral patients for the tertiary center, and services and subsidies for the outlying facilities. As the networks develop, the primary benefits will be (1) managed care contracts that protect market share for all hospitals and physicians, and (2) the economies of operation from a fully integrated delivery system.

The "alliance" can be a model for the regional delivery system of the 1990s. Milwaukee's Horizon Healthcare is a "non-ownership alliance" of three area hospitals launched in 1989. Executives and board members came together to collaborate on managed care initiatives and clinical programs. Governance is shared equally. Each partner has an equal voice in voting, representation, and decision making. The alliance-based system works, says Robert Drisner, CEO of Community Memorial Hospital: "We didn't see a need [for a merger] because the way Horizon is structured certainly meets all the criteria of an integrated system without the consolidation of assets. I don't think it would have been possible to bring together three very strong independent organizations and boards" (Anderson 1992).

The network is the independent hospital's response to the "Super-Meds" prediction that all hospitals would be owned by very large national systems. That never happened. A slim majority—51%—of the nation's 7,000 hospitals currently belong to multi-hospital systems, according to the American Hospital Association.

Instead, hospitals adopted the network, or "consortia," model, and began building systems through voluntary affiliation and alliance. The network model will be the dominant pattern of hospital-physician relations in the 1990s.

The affiliations and alliances of a successful hub-and-spoke network rely on locally specific mutual benefit. Most networks give small hospitals access to group purchasing contracts, which can provide savings of 10 to 40 percent on supplies and equipment. Some networks also make group purchasing available to the hospital's physicians. Other services include management contracting, clinical department contracting, physician education, staff recruitment, accounting and information systems, quality assurance, licensing and certification compliance, marketing and planning, and shared advertising. Even a new CEO or chief financial officer can be part of the package. Some networks provide loaned executives on a short- or long-term basis.

In return for patient referrals, hub medical centers can provide capital, facilities, and equipment to the smaller network hospitals. One such medical center is building medical office buildings on the campuses of affiliated hospitals, which will include support services such as radiology, laboratory, diagnostic, corporate health, psychology, and pharmacy. Many networks support group practice development, some also manage small medical groups, and a few networks have purchased medical practices. The goal is to create an integrated regional service distribution system that will outcompete other local hospitals for insurance and managed care contracts.

The network concept is appealing. It is relatively simple to construct and requires little capital. But the affiliation concept has a serious weakness: its reliance on voluntary cooperation. Basically a network is a confederation; commitment by local hospitals to cooperate with the decisions and directions of the network is completely voluntary.

If every decision is open to challenge, and every managed care contract needs validation by all network members, then the network can rapidly fall apart. A spirit of trust by local hospital members is essential to continued cohesion, along with a form of governance consistent with the alliance model of voluntary affiliation. Perhaps the best governance of networks will be by mutual cooperation at the trustee level—a "council of allies." Participating hospitals will send delegates to the network's regional council. Strategic decisions will be collaborative. But ultimately, the majority must rule and partners must commit to the network decision. If voluntary networks fail, more integrated models—including a government takeover—may follow.

Strategy 3. Centers of Excellence and Clinical Networks

The centerpieces of American hospital market strategy today are medical centers of excellence—cardiac care, oncology, obstetrics, and other specialized services. The market pull of these "magnet" services must be reinforced by the creation of clinical networks, which reach out to referring hospitals and physicians. In the future, centers of excellence will provide an opportunity to contract for "bundled" physician-hospital services, such as the package of specialized procedures involved in cardiac arterial bypass grafts. Or centers of excellence may subcapitate, for instance, for orthopedic services, contracting with an HMO or employer for all patients who need specialty care.

Clinical networks formalize and give structure to traditionally informal patterns of medical referral. There are benefits to all parties. Tertiary hospitals provide specialized physician services to outlying hospitals, allowing local patients to receive consulting services at home without leaving the community. Some specialized clinical networks develop written protocols for patient referral and transfer, specifying the communication, privileges, and guarantees of patient return to reassure local doctors.

A national network of cancer centers was formed by 13 of the nation's best-known oncology programs, including Memorial Sloan-Kettering Medical Center in New York, M. D. Anderson in Houston, and Stanford University in California (Japsen 1995). Through the network called the National Comprehensive Cancer Network, the hospitals hope to attract the nation's largest employers and managed care plans. As a network of premier oncology programs, the cancer centers believe their sustained competitive advantage will be the cost-effective management of complex cancer care. The network plans to assess new methods of cancer treatments, in terms of costs and effectiveness. All centers share an information network and database and have already developed local hub-and-spoke cancer networks in their marketplaces.

Clinical networks are "bridge" strategies to more extensive alliances and partnerships. Clinical networks among hospitals and physicians are an excellent training ground for collaboration. They can build a base of trust for managed care networking and even merger.

Strategy 4. Primary Care Networks

To succeed in tomorrow's managed care, managed competition marketplace, every hospital and system needs a primary care base. Hospital boards need to rethink fundamentally their capital investment strategy, redirecting capital into physician acquisition, group practice development, and ambulatory facilities for primary care both on and off campus.

The reason is simple: HMOs and insurers rely on primary care physicians to be gatekeepers to the healthcare system and to take responsibility as integrators of care instead of third-party review organizations. There are four strategies for constructing primary care networks (Engstrom 1995):

Split primary care and specialists. Organizers can focus on recruiting primary care physicians and contract for specialty care separately. In Eugene, the Oregon Medical Group is made up exclusively of 52 primary care physicians, including several obstetrician/gynecologists. The group has resisted heated suggestions to add subspecialists and has even lobbied sponsoring Sacred Heart Hospital against hiring four surgeons.

Organize in two phases. Organizers can begin with a core of primary care physicians and let them choose which specialists should be invited to join the group, as did the Premier Medical Group in Denver. As in Eugene, however, controversy is likely to follow when specialists protest their exclusion.

Start with multispecialty and add primary. When most of the medical community are specialists, networks may start with a multispecialty group and diversify into primary care, as have the Carle Clinic in Urbana, Illinois, and the Fargo Clinic in North Dakota.

Combine primary IPA and multispecialty clinic. Organizing a primary care–oriented independent practice association can complement an established multispecialty group practice, such as the Lutheran General Health Plan, now Advocate Health, which combines a 270-doctor multispecialty clinic with a 600-physician IPA.

Strategy 5. Managing Quality

Far-sighted physicians have long seen the need for managing medical and hospital quality. Governance consultant James Orlikoff reaches back to 1916, citing one of America's pioneers in medical outcomes, Dr. E. A. Codman, on the importance of managing quality (Orlikoff 1993):

I am called eccentric for saying in public that hospitals, if they wish to be sure of improvement:

- Must find out what their results are.

- Must analyze their results to find their strong and weak points.
- Must compare their results with those of other hospitals.
- Must care for what cases they can care for well, and avoid attempting to care for cases which they are not qualified to care for well.
- Must welcome publicity not only for their successes but for their errors, so that the public may give them their help when it is needed.
- Must promote members of the medical staff on the basis which gives due consideration to what they can and do accomplish for their patients.

Dr. Codman noted that "such opinions will not be eccentric a few years hence." He was right, but it took another 75 years. The time for managing quality is now. Quality becomes a critical success factor in a marketplace where purchasers have detailed clinical data on the outcomes of hospital and physician performance.

Physicians must review quality performance using a set of key clinical indicators. Orlikoff (1993) suggests that the hospital regularly review such factors as:

- mortality rates (e.g., overall hospitalwide mortality rate, neonatal and maternal mortality rate, surgical mortality rate);
- nosocomial infection rates (e.g., overall hospitalwide nosocomial infection rate, postoperative infection rate);
- adverse drug reactions or interactions;
- unplanned returns to surgery;
- unplanned transfers to surgery, isolation, intensive care, or cardiac care units;
- unplanned transfers to other acute care facilities;
- hospital-incurred traumas;
- discharges against medical advice;
- returns to the emergency room within 72 hours of being treated in the ER;
- readmissions to the hospital within one month of discharge;
- unplanned admissions to the hospital following outpatient procedures; and
- cesarean-section rates.

Physician-hospital "economic organizations" such as independent practice associations—not the organized medical staff—may ultimately take lead responsibility for credentialing physicians and managing physician quality. Medical consultant Daniel A. Lang, M.D., predicts that peer review will increasingly be affected by external requirements, and the organized medical staff may no longer be the locus of peer review (Ewell 1993). Dr. Lang notes that economic organizations, including PHOs and IPAs, will decide which physicians will be part of the medical group that shares managed care contracts with the hospital.

HMOs, hospitals, doctors, and health systems will compete on the basis of quality. Sophisticated purchasers, insurance plans, self-insured employers, and governments will all have detailed data on quality performance. In California, a statewide "report card" has compared the quality of care between 15 HMOs (Sanders 1995). Four health plans won high marks, but three others were faulted as "below average." The report was prepared by the California Cooperative HEDIS Reporting Initiative, a coalition of HMOs, employers, and physician groups. The report utilizes a database of quality indicators such as childhood immunizations, cholesterol screenings, and prenatal care.

Hospitals and their medical staffs and physician organizations need to develop jointly a comprehensive ongoing system for auditing quality. Then hospitals can use their quality improvement processes systematically to improve quality, in terms of both clinical care and customer satisfaction.

BUILDING A CULTURE OF HOSPITAL-PHYSICIAN COOPERATION

The most important finding from a national study of the hospital-physician relationship is the importance of a *culture* that emphasizes board and management working jointly with physicians in pursuing the institution's mission and objectives (Shortell 1991). As John Yorty, chairman of the Estes Park Institute, notes, "There is nothing more important to the successful operation of a hospital than a medical staff that works in harmony with the hospital. And there is nothing more difficult to attain and maintain" (Shortell et al. 1993).

Shortell has developed a "stage model" of hospital-physician relationships that outlines the evolution of a culture of trust and collaboration (see Table 9.1). A culture of physician-hospital collaboration is required by environmental changes, argues Harvard's Alan Sheldon, "yet if it is trivial, it is meaningless" (Sheldon 1979). Significant physician-hospital cooperative effort requires

Table 9.1
A Stage Model of Hospital-Physician Relationships

Stages	Characteristics	Requirements for Effectiveness
Stage I Early (Infancy)	Low experience Low capabilities Low confidence	Strong culture Strong board Extensive education Develop relationship fundamentals High outside consultation Some early successes
Stage II Middle (Adolescence)	Some experience Some capabilities Moderate confidence (sometimes misplaced)	Understanding board Patient administration Willingness to experiment Ability to accept failure Learn from mistakes Continued education Some trust builders
Stage III Late (Maturity)	High experience High capabilities High confidence	Facilitating board Shared management and governance Build on successes Seek new opportunities Continued education Avoid complacency Shared some failures

Source: Shortell, S. M. Effective Hospital-Physician Relationships. © 1991. Reprinted with permission from the Hospital Research and Educational Trust.

"paradigm-breaking" effort, which is why collaboration has proven to be so difficult and poorly handled. Most hospital executives recognized the need for significant physician involvement in the mid-1980s, and a new era of "conjoint" physician-hospital effort began (Shortell 1990).

The successes of the 10 hospitals and health systems profiled in Shortell's study is inspiring. But it would be a mistake to ignore the impediments and failures that often occurred. Trust between board, administration, and medical staff was a critical success factor. Often this trust was built upon long-developed personal relationships between the board, senior management, and medical staff leadership. Most of the CEOs in the study hospitals had five to ten years of experience in the facility, with strong board continuity.

The ten-hospital study searched for and found cross-cutting strategies that promoted a climate of trust for physician-hospital collaboration. To achieve successful hospital-physician relations, hospitals must effectively manage six key issues: (1) physician-hospital competition, (2) managed care, (3) joint ventures, (4) cost containment, (5) nurse-physician relationships, and (6) quality improvement.

As hospital boards and their medical staffs face the future, they need a process of shared decision making and governance. From a process perspective, here are the secrets of effective physician-hospital relationships:

- open decision-making and managerial style;
- extensive physician involvement;
- continuous communication;
- mutual trust;
- a process for resolving conflict; and
- willingness to change.

CAUSES OF MEDICAL STAFF–ADMINISTRATION BREAKDOWN

Physician-hospital relationships are among the most important "make-break" factors in a hospital's success—and in CEO survival. Creating a partnership for governance of tomorrow's integrated health systems will not be easy, cautions healthcare consultant and futurist Jeff Goldsmith: "Both sides of the bizarre, sadomasochist relationship between medical practice and management bring baggage to the 'arranged marriage' of the integrated healthcare system" (Goldsmith 1993).

Generations of physician leaders have sought to preserve clinical autonomy and entrepreneurship, but the emerging marketplace of managed care and integrated systems encourages sharing of power and collegiality. Doctors are trained as independent decision makers. Goldsmith argues that doctors will make "terrible employees—ask any medical school dean or group practice CEO." What is needed is hospital-physician collegiality, which must be based on tolerance and the sharing of common professional values. In turbulent times, the trust relationship between management and medical staff undergoes heavy stress. A national survey on U.S. hospitals and the future by Deloitte & Touche (1992) found that hospital-physician relationships were not as compatible in 1992 as they were four years earlier in a previous survey. Only 31 percent of hospital CEOs characterized their relationships with physicians as "excellent" in 1992, down from 37 percent.

Both sides are to blame. Here are five key reasons why healthcare executives get in trouble with their medical staffs:

Withholding strategic information. Often this problem is labeled "communication." What the doctors really mean is that top administration likes to operate from an information advantage, and key information is either late or incomplete when it is presented to the medical staff.

Hospital-physician competition. As hospitals expand their ambulatory care activities, they begin to compete very directly with the two-thirds of the medical staff who are office-based practitioners. Equipment wars are a variation on the theme of competition, when the hospital acquires technology such as magnetic resonance imaging, which competes with physician-owned equipment.

"Bonding" backlash. When hospitals employ a variety of incentives to strengthen their ties with key admitters, other physicians are likely to feel neglected or threatened. Their feelings are real and often justified.

Weak (or hostile) medical staff leadership. Failure of medical staff leadership to lead or communicate is a frequent cause of the disintegration of trust between medical staff and administration. Worse yet, some immature medical staffs deliberately choose a weak or antagonistic doctor to represent them.

Lack of shared incentives. An underlying problem in most hospitals is the lack of shared incentives between doctors and the hospital, with a handful of exceptions like Kaiser, Henry Ford, and the Mayo Clinic. Hospitals are now paid primarily by case or stay, while doctors are still reimbursed fee-for-service. Only in risk-sharing arrangements with managed care plans do physicians and management share economic incentives for efficiency. Until this problem is solved, hospitals and their doctors will only cooperate based on good will and a concern for quality patient care.

The physician culture is fundamentally different from the culture shared by board and management, argues Martin D. Merry, M.D., professor of health management and policy at the University of New Hampshire. The board and management believe leadership includes vision, strategy, communications, and consensus building. The doctors have other ideas. The physician culture, Dr. Merry suggests, believes leaders should

- Be clinically competent.
- Carry out certain bylaw provisions relating to accreditation and facilitate a peer review process to ensure quality.

- Advise administration on technology and other practice needs.
- Represent physicians' interests to administration and the board. Possibly greatest among these interests is the felt need for personal autonomy unencumbered by the bureaucratic rules that seem to govern most institutions. (Merry 1993)

Physicians who are admired as leaders by their colleagues are those who are first and foremost clinically excellent. Strong physician leaders do not build consensus. They build excellent clinical programs. Physician leaders do not build support for institutional vision, or risk being considered "administrative stooges" for promoting the "hospital's agenda." The physician culture does not build team players. The independent thinking so essential for clinical decision making is at odds with an organizational culture of group decisions and teamwork.

Dr. Merry (1993) predicts two types of physician leaders will emerge: those who make the full transition to true healthcare executives and those who divide their time between patient care and administrative duties. Such part-time physician leaders will be critical to physician-hospital integration in this transitional period, while hospitals and systems develop the medically trained healthcare executives for the future.

WHEN PHYSICIAN LEADERSHIP DOES NOT REPRESENT THE RANK-AND-FILE

Physician-hospital integration is a rocky road, littered with the debris of failed projects and fired executives. Too often, the problem has been that the physician "rank-and-file" did not buy in to a proposal agreed upon by its own medical leadership. Managing an integrated healthcare organization requires widespread physician participation in decision making at all levels of the organization.

Without broad support from practicing physicians, new physician-hospital initiatives will be vulnerable to apathy, slow implementation, and even sabotage from the medical staff. Weak or isolated medical leadership is often to blame. According to one physician leader, "You have to understand that we are really three groups—the management and board, the medical staff leadership, and the rank-and-file. For the most part, we (the medical staff leadership) are much closer to management and the board than we are to the rank and file" (Shortell 1991).

The split between medical staff leaders and the rank-and-file is a common issue in many medical staffs where the leadership represents older physicians with well-established practices, versus many younger medical staff members who are working 60 to 70 hours a week to build a practice. These younger physicians in the Shortell study expressed general suspicion of the hospital as an institution, a wariness of medical staff leadership, and a "show me" attitude. Apathy often prevailed unless these alienated physicians could see the direct relevance of a hospital decision to their own practices. One hospital's attempt to establish a medical director position was frustrated when the medical staff voted 67 to 59 to censure the medical staff executive committee for proposing the position. The "no" vote shocked the medical leadership, who had polled the 150 physicians on the medical staff earlier on the issue of recruiting a medical director, and found two-thirds in favor (Shortell 1991).

SHARED GOVERNANCE FOR REAL PHYSICIAN-HOSPITAL PARTNERSHIPS

If the goal is to change the way healthcare is delivered in the community, everyone in the physician community must be heard. When CEOs and other hospital executives begin to contemplate the development of networks, they need to ask physicians for their input. They must get every physician's opinion, especially the opinion of those physicians who compete directly against them or who complain the loudest (Daugherty 1993).

The underlying reality is that only about one-third of the medical staff really need the hospital. The rest of the medical staff is office-based. New and better physician strategies are needed that are based on the long-term interdependence of hospitals with physicians. The pressure is rising. Malpractice liability and financial risk will be shared. Managed care and government regulations are forcing hospital-physician collaboration, whether all parties are ready or not.

What is needed is a new emphasis on teamwork and collaboration. Hospital advisor Don L. Arnwine calls on the board to take leadership in teamwork: "Although the board members aren't responsible for selecting and evaluating individual members of the CEO's senior team, they should take a keen interest in how the group is functioning. . . . The board should make sure that incentives are tied equally to team accomplishments and individual performance" (Arnwine 1992).

Arnwine's survey of dozens of U.S. hospitals and health systems makes some key points with regard to the challenges of collaboration and a team approach:

- Chief executives have a consistently more positive view of team performance than team members themselves.
- Team members and CEOs share a high level of optimism.
- Fatigue and lack of family time are viewed as significant problems.
- Making decisions efficiently is the biggest challenge.
- Lack of communication often clouds the common agenda.
- Teams worry about how they are viewed by employees and the medical staff. (Arnwine 1992)

Board support of a team concept between management and the medical staff can reinforce a shared optimism and a positive outlook toward the challenges of managing a modern hospital or health system. Open communication and a common agenda are critical to success. The sense of team and collaborative spirit must permeate the entire organization, beginning with the board and senior management team, and spreading across the employees and medical staff. Shared vision, high levels of performance, and achievement of desired outcomes can result from strong teams.

PHYSICIAN-HOSPITAL COMPUTER LINKAGES

Healthcare, high technology, computers, and medicine—what could seem a more natural combination for hospitals in the "Information Age"? Physician-computer linkages have been in place in dozens of hospitals for more than five years, and a growing number of hospitals are developing them. The promise of these linkages is the rapid transmission of data between the hospital and the doctor's office. The goal is to reinforce the symbolic connection between a hospital and its key admitters, enhance quality patient care through expedited data transmission, and position physicians to manage care and costs under capitation. To date, however, costs are high, and benefits are limited.

Satisfaction with health information systems is only "so-so," according to a 1995 survey (Bergman 1995). Less than half of the respondents (48 percent) report being satisfied with their information system products, and 11 percent are definitely dissatisfied. West Coast providers are least happy (40 percent are not satisfied with the current information system), because their applications do not effectively support provider networks in a capitated marketplace.

Despite provider skepticism, computer-link systems do work, and data are flowing for laboratory results, radiology results, insurance and billing, pharmacy results, census information, and admissions data. Comparing two surveys, by 1994 the number of hospital-physician computer links was not substantially higher, and the range of data shared had not broadened significantly (Bergman 1995). Both physician offices and hospitals have achieved high levels of computerization, but their systems stand side-by-side, with little effective interaction. There is widespread disappointment with the systems' limited applications and technological bugs. Further, physician acceptance of physician-link systems has been slow.

It is too early for systems to deliver the full potential of linking a doctor's office with a hospital's information system. Hospitals should not expect dramatic results from their linkage systems in terms of increased admissions or better physician information on costs or quality. These will come as hardware gets cheaper, software becomes more user-friendly, and the available information from the system expands. The 1980s were a time for innovators and early adapters. By the year 2000, more than 90 percent of all hospitals over 200 beds will have installed computer linkages in the offices of their key physicians and medical groups. Doctors and hospitals will be symbiotically linked. Computer linkage systems will be the ties that bind them together.

PAYING FOR INTEGRATION STRATEGIES

Healthcare finance consultant Ronald Barkley (1995) asks the capital question regarding integration strategies: "You've done it all! You merged three hospitals, partnered with a large multispecialty medical group, linked with a geographically dispersed primary care network/IPA, and negotiated a 50/50 joint venture with a strong regional HMO. You're looking like an integrated delivery system and you're the envy of your colleagues. Now, how are you going to pay for it all?"

The amount of capital required to pursue integration strategies could be substantial. In a survey on the capital needs of emerging healthcare organizations (Barkley 1995), a sample of 500 provider groups identified a potential need for $1 billion to fund integration efforts in the next two to three years. More specifically, capital needs projections averaged:

- independent practice associations and managed care networks—$1.2 million;
- physician-hospital organizations—$2.2 million;
- management service networks—$9.6 million;
- freestanding medical groups—$19.7 million; and
- foundation models—$20 million.

Barkley identifies a range of innovative sources of startup and development capital that are available for emerging integrated entities:

Letter of credit or commercial paper. An existing organization with little equity but a strong cash flow, such as a physician group, may find working with a sophisticated commercial bank provides quick access to funds without the need for personal guarantees by participating doctors.

Deferred compensation. A source of internal capital can be deferred compensation, which can, for example, be escrowed as the medical group participants' share of an eighty-twenty loan for construction of a medical office.

Share of the equity. Another vehicle for raising capital can be selling a minority or majority share in the partners' equity, such as to an insurance company, health system, or entrepreneurial company such as Phycor or CareMark.

Taxable commercial paper. For an established organization that may own a medical group, HMO, or hospital assets, use of taxable commerical paper taps into the deep capital pockets of large institutional investors, including pension funds and insurance companies. Healthcare borrowers may need a bank of letter of credit to obtain investment-grade credit ratings.

For-profit and nonprofit joint venture. An innovative source of capital for nonprofit providers may be to sell hospital assets to a for-profit corporation, such as Columbia/HCA. The nonprofit providers maintain partial control of the organization by reinvesting the sale proceeds in the joint venture.

LOOKING FORWARD: FIVE STRATEGIES FOR STRENGTHENING THE PARTNERSHIP

Here are five promising approaches to developing a strong, committed relationship between a hospital and its key physicians.

1. *Physician-hospital organization.* Leadership can reconstruct relationships between the hospital and physicians to establish an integrated physician-hospital organization. The PHO can jointly contract with managed care plans as a hospitalwide organization. In a completely integrated model, all members of the active medical staff join together in a professional corporation covering all clinical departments. This group-model arrangement is sometimes

called the Kaiser model, from the relationship between the Kaiser Foundation Health Plan (hospitals) and the Kaiser Permanente Medical Group (physicians). An integrated model is essential regardless of the form of national health reform. The healthcare market will demand regional delivery systems of hospitals and physicians who can contract with managed care insurance plans and self-insured employers to carry out specified patient care, quality assurance, and cost management activities.

2. *Vice president for medical care.* A doctor should be placed in charge of the doctors. This senior management position needs to have full authority and responsibility for the medical care provided in the hospital. Like the chief engineer in a manufacturing organization or the chief scientist in a high-technology firm, the vice president for medical care will plan, organize, direct, and control medical care in the hospital. The person in this position should be a voting member (an "inside" director) of the board of trustees. Reporting to this vice president, chiefs of clinical services and medical directors of programs will have direct line responsibility for their medical care provided within their departments.

3. *Physicians in governance.* The hospital's board of directors should include substantial physician representation. Between one-third (33 percent) and, preferably, one-half (49 percent) of the board should be doctors. Physicians should regularly chair major committees such as finance and planning, and rotate as chair of the board of trustees. Boards need more clinical expertise and physician input for success in the 1990s. Physicians must be an integral part of the management and governance of the hospital and health system at every level.

4. *Clinical management.* The successful hospital is clinically efficient and effective. Its goals are top-quality service at the lowest feasible cost per case, per stay, and per procedure. Financial success is dependent upon fine-tuning the clinical management that controls costs for every patient and service. The medical management challenge will be to coordinate case management, utilization review, quality assurance, and traditional clinical aspects with cost control, staffing, and support services. This is why hospital boards need substantial physician participation—to understand and manage the core business of clinical care.

5. *Integrated information systems.* Hospitals in the 1990s will live or die based on the quality of their data systems. Physician and nurse case managers must have the ability to manage their patients in real time. Financial and clinical data must be timely and accurate. Computerized workstations should be networked and universally accessible across the hospital, ambulatory settings, and physician

offices. The fine-tuning of clinical management could save the average hospital at least one-half to one full patient day. Quicker, more accurate diagnoses and more efficient use of resources during the stay or procedure may add 3 to 5 percent to the hospital's bottom line. The board of trustees should regularly review a set of key medical performance indicators on the hospital's clinical cost-efficiency and quality. Hospitals must catch up with other U.S. businesses in the effectiveness of their information systems. Hospitals should strengthen their board composition with trustee expertise in information systems.

STRATEGIC IMPLICATIONS FOR PROVIDERS, HMOs, AND SUPPLIERS

Providers

The next phase in hospital-physician relations will be determined by the "culture of cooperation" that Shortell (1991) recommends. Integrated provider networks must be open to medical viewpoints, and physician leadership must be substantially involved in governance. Hospitals and health systems need to increase their efforts to strengthen the practices of their physicians and develop effective organizations (IPAs, MSOs, HMOs) to give their doctors access to managed care contracts. Every hospital of more than 150 beds, and every multihospital system, should have a full-time physician executive who is a member of the senior management group and who also sits as a trustee on the board. The vice president for medical care needs to be integrally involved in hospital policymaking and leadership at the highest level.

HMOs

Provider integration is both a threat and an opportunity for HMOs, insurers, and third party payers. Development of integrated delivery networks and physician-hospital organizations positions providers for at-risk contracting. These are the building blocks for provider-sponsored HMOs and direct contracting, a serious competitive threat. Alternatively, provider integration may create the groundwork for a closer, multi-year, and even exclusive contractual relationship between providers and health plans. On a long-term basis, HMOs must recognize that their competitive position in the food chain is dependent upon the performance of the underlying provider network. In other words, the provider network "is the HMO" to patients and purchasers. This may create the basis for new synergies between providers and payers.

Suppliers

There are two important consequences for suppliers resulting from physician-hospital integration. First, hospitals and doctors are no longer "two customers." The integration of providers will consolidate purchasing decisions and increase the level of physician influence in cost management. Second, the increased emphasis on disease management and clinical pathways will have major consequences for the consumption of supplies, equipment, and patient care materials. Suppliers should pursue business partner strategies and share development activities, such as product development and clinical trials, with preferred networks of providers.

SOURCES

Anderson, H. 1992. "Hospitals Seek New Ways to Integrate Health Care." *Hospitals.* 66 (7): 26–36

Arnwine, D. L. 1992. *The Power of Teamwork in an Age of Collaboration.* La Jolla, CA: The Governance Institute.

Barkley, R. 1995. "How Are You Going to Pay for It?" *Integrated Healthcare Report* (November): 1–8.

Bergman, R. 1995. "Stone Age Solutions: IS Vendors Aren't Keeping Pace with Today's Delivery Needs." *Hospitals & Health Networks* 69 (3): 27–32.

Cochrane, J. 1995. "PacifiCare Completes First Phase of Provider Stock Ownership Incentive Plan." *Integrated Healthcare Report* (November): 19.

Codman, E. A. 1916. *A Study in Hospital Efficiency*, cited by James E. Orlikoff, "Involving Hospital Trustees in the Quality Management Process." Presentation at the Hospital Medical Staff and Trustee Conference, The Governance Institute, Maui, Hawaii, January 12, 1993.

Coile, Jr., R. C. 1994. "Capitation: The New 'Food Chain' of HMO-Provider Payment." *Hospital Strategy Report* 6 (9): 1–8.

Daugherty, M. L. 1993. "Involve Doctors in Building Networks." *Modern Healthcare* 23 (14): 29.

Deloitte & Touche. 1992. *U.S. Hospitals and the Future of Health Care: A Continuing Opinion Survey.* Boston, MA: Deloitte & Touche.

Engstrom, P. 1995. "Medical Group Practices Need More Than Luck in the Provider-Mix Game." *Medical Network Strategy Report* 4 (2): 1–3.

Ewell, C. 1993. "Medical Leadership Institute Offered Practical Tools and Techniques for a Changing Environment." *Medical Leadership Press* 1 (6): 1–5.

Glatstein, H. R. 1993. "Physician Organizational Formation." Presentation to the Physician Leadership Conference, Legacy Health System, Portland, Oregon, April 3.

Goldsmith, J. 1993. "Driving the Nitroglycerin Truck." *Healthcare Forum Journal* 2 (36): 36–44.

Japsen, B. 1995. "Cancer Network's Goal: Draw Business." *Modern Healthcare* 25 (6): 20.

Johnsson, J. 1992. "Dynamic Diversification: Hospitals Pursue Physician Alliances, 'Seamless' Care." *Hospitals* 66 (3): 20–26.

Kaufman, N. 1995. "Strategy: Power Notebook." *Hospitals & Health Systems* 69 (3): 58–62.

McKemy, V. 1995. "Doctors May Play a Bigger Leadership Role in Networks of the Future." *Medical Network Strategy Report* 4 (2): 10–12.

Merry, M. D. 1993. *Understanding How Physician Leaders Think*. La Jolla, CA: The Governance Institute.

Norling, R. 1995. "Baptism by Fire." *Hospitals & Health Networks* 69 (3): 50.

Orlikoff, J. E. 1993. "Involving Hospital Trustees in the Quality Management Process." Presentation at the Hospital Medical Staff and Trustee Conference, The Governance Institute, Maui, Hawaii, January 12.

Rudd, T. 1995. "Indirect Physician Links Fuel Columbia/HCA's Houston Strategy." *Healthcare Systems Strategy Report* 12 (3): 12

Sanders, E. "HMO Checkup: Study Rates Quality of Care Given in State," *Los Angeles Daily News*, 23 February 1995, p. B1.

Sheldon, A. 1979. *Managing Change and Collaboration in the Health System*. Cambridge, MA: Oelgeschlager, Gunn & Hain.

Shortell, S. M. 1991. *Effective Hospital-Physician Relationships*. Ann Arbor, MI: Health Administration Press.

———. 1990. "The Medical Staff of the Future: Replanting the Garden." *Frontiers of Health Services Management* 7 (1): 3–48.

Shortell, S. M., D. A. Anderson, R. R. Gillies, J. B. Mitchell, K. L. Morgan. 1993 "The Holographic Organization." *Healthcare Forum Journal* 36 (2): 20–28.

Sokolov, J. J. 1993. "On the Brink of a Third Generation." *Healthcare Forum Journal* 36 (2): 29–33.

CHAPTER 10

Provider-Payer Partnerships: Creating the Ultimate Model

The ultimate survivor may be the product of fully merging the insurer/HMO, hospital system and medical group functions . . . a system that takes advantage of the strengths of each and minimizes issues of power and dominance . . . a system that is strongly driven by the direct care givers—the physicians at the core.

John Cochrane (1993a, 8)

A GRAND ALLIANCE between providers and payers will develop into fully integrated health systems for the twenty-first century. Hospitals and medical groups should move now to choose their insurer and HMO partners. Providers must organize to create exclusive relationships with insurers. Providers must assume that the future will be an HMO, and that they will have only three choices: build or buy equity stakes in an HMO; become a partner in joint business relationships with HMOs; or be a vendor to HMOs, on their terms.

The two most powerful forces pushing toward payer-provider partnerships are: (1) managed care and capitation; and (2) market reform, demanded by cost-conscious employers. What the market wants and health reform seeks is cost-effective integration between providers and payers. Purchasers—whether they are major employers, state Medicaid programs, or business coalitions—must drive down HMO administrative costs to 6 to 8 percent and

Five Stages of Managed Care

restrain healthcare price inflation to 3 to 4 percent per year, in line with the consumer price index. Hospitals need HMO and insurer partnerships to give them preferred access to covered lives.

In searching for managed care partners, hospitals should look first at HMOs. Health maintenance organizations are making a strong move to overtake insurers as the dominant payment plans. The number of HMO enrollees reached 50 million in 1994 (see Fig. 10.1), according to the Group Health Association of America (Palsbo 1994). HMOs are now growing at an annual rate of 9 to 10 percent per year, and employers like HMO prices. While conventional health insurance prices have been rising, HMOs cut their premiums in 1995 for the fifth straight year (Sardinha 1994).

WHO WILL WIN? INSURERS AND HMOs OR HOSPITALS AND PHYSICIANS?

The biggest question to be answered about the creation of the ultimate system model is: Who owns the networks? Will deep-pocketed insurers and HMOs simply acquire or rent providers? Or can hospitals and medical groups develop strong regional delivery systems that "rent" the insurance function? Or will all parties agree to a business alliance on a partnership model to create the ultimate system? Here are the options for control of the networks and the post-reform managed care marketplace:

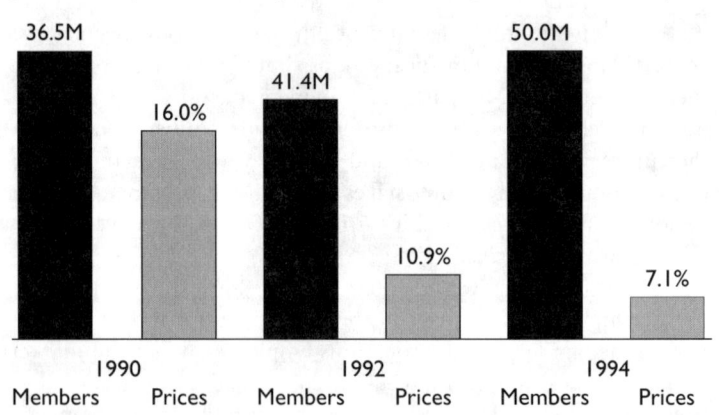

Figure 10.1 HMO Membership and Prices, 1990–94 (membership in millions, prices in percentage annual increase)

1990		1992		1994	
Members	Prices	Members	Prices	Members	Prices
36.5M	16.0%	41.4M	10.9%	50.0M	7.1%

Source: Adapted from Susan E. Palsbo, Group Health Association of America, Washington, D.C., 1994.

Insurers and HMOs. Insurers and HMOs are the most obvious winners in organizing networks. They hold the customers, have the capital resources, and can simply acquire the providers or contract with them at a discount. With the surplus of hospitals and physicians in most local regions, this is a buyer's market that favors the insurers and HMOs. In the long run, the organization farthest up the reimbursement stream, the one with most control of enrollees and premium dollars, will deal from a position of strength. But the market is insisting on lower administrative costs from insurers and HMOs, which the health plans cannot deliver without provider cooperation.

Hospitals and health systems. In many local markets, hospitals provide the nucleus and the energy for the creation of regional provider networks. Across the country, hospitals and health systems are constructing multihospital business alliances for managed care contracting. The hub-and-spoke model features dominant regional medical centers or teaching hospitals. A high-reputation hospital can make its market and choose its HMO and insurer partners. Hubless systems keep their infrastructure costs down by contracting out-of-network for tertiary services. Hospitals must be network organizers, or they will be vendors to insurers and HMOs that contract for beds at substantial per diem discounts.

Medical groups. The power of primary care–oriented physician groups is growing. Recognizing their potential, large medical group practices are taking global capitation contracts from HMOs and insurers and subcontracting with hospitals and outside specialists for a comprehensive service package. As the medical groups grow, they can add physicians, construct a multisite delivery network, contract with hospitals at favorable per diem rates, and even purchase their own hospitals. Equity in physician-owned networks gives doctors an opportunity to regain financial and clinical control of their practices. The odds for success may be long—physicians are handicapped by lack of management, capital, and such infrastructure as care protocols and information networks—but these medical groups own the doctors, who are the ultimate success factor in any model.

THE MANAGED CARE TRIAD

Under capitation, the key players of the managed care triad (see Fig. 10.2)—HMOs and insurers, hospitals, and physicians—will restructure relationships to consolidate costs. Under capitation, the duplication and redundancy of market competition will be luxuries that increase costs and cut into the profits that all three parties

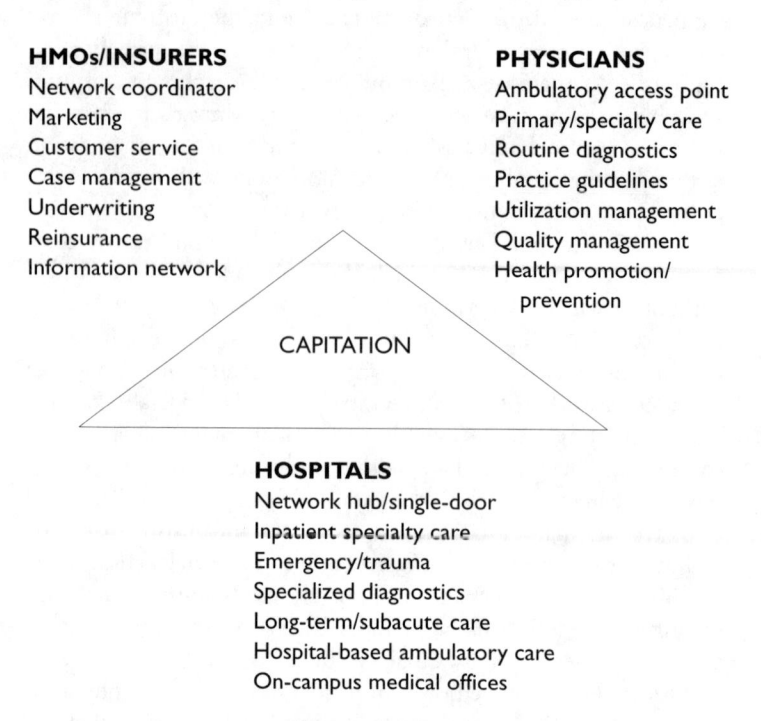

Figure 10.2 The Rationalizing Roles of the Managed Care Triad

HMOs/INSURERS
Network coordinator
Marketing
Customer service
Case management
Underwriting
Reinsurance
Information network

PHYSICIANS
Ambulatory access point
Primary/specialty care
Routine diagnostics
Practice guidelines
Utilization management
Quality management
Health promotion/
   prevention

CAPITATION

HOSPITALS
Network hub/single-door
Inpatient specialty care
Emergency/trauma
Specialized diagnostics
Long-term/subacute care
Hospital-based ambulatory care
On-campus medical offices

Source: Coile, Jr., R. C. 1995. "Managed Care Outlook 1995–2000." Health Trends 7 (5): 1–8.

share. Duplicated programs, such as open-heart surgery, will be recognized as internal competition and consolidated. All players will share the incentives to reduce or eliminate excess capacity, unneeded care, and administrative expenses.

Hospitals and health systems will build hub-and-spoke networks of care settings, with comprehensive continuums from critical care to ambulatory and long-term care. Acute care hospitals will become 300-bed intensive care units. Nonacute patients will be treated in ambulatory, long-term, or home settings, reducing hospital days by 25 to 35 percent. Hospitals will downsize or close excess beds to reduce inpatient costs, and eliminate duplication of functions. High-overhead services like trauma and cardiac surgery will be regionalized. Physicians and nurses will collaborate on clinical treatment protocols to optimize efficiency. The cost-reduction potential could shrink the hospital component of the capitated premium from 38 to 40 percent to 30 to 32 percent.

Medical groups will provide patient care, including primary and specialty medicine, manage clinical costs, develop treatment protocols, and monitor quality and outcomes. Primary care–based multispecialty groups will be preferred partners for HMOs and hospital networks. Specialists will expand single-specialty groups and build regional specialty networks for selective contracting, for example, for obstetrics, orthopedics, or urology. Specialty groups will bid for volume contracts on specific procedures like transurethral resections, cataracts, and hip replacements. Fewer outpatients will be scheduled for return visits, and physicians will exercise greater restraint in ordering tests and procedures. Doctors will reduce overhead by consolidating practices into fewer sites. Medical office buildings will be built for group practice. Doctors will be paid a salary, plus incentives for group performance. Ambulatory care centers staffed by primary care physicians and nurse practitioners will provide urgent care, reducing emergency room demand by 60 to 75 percent and ER costs by 40 to 50 percent. Despite the need for capital investment to fund ambulatory expansion, the overall cost savings in ambulatory care due to increased physician efficiency and reduced overhead could be in the range of 15 to 25 percent.

Insurers and HMOs will provide marketing, customer relations, finance, information systems, and network coordination. Once HMOs put providers under capitation, they can slash overhead costs for utilization management and third-party review. Reducing provider management costs could boost HMO and insurer profits by 30 to 50 percent. But strong medical groups and high-reputation hospital networks will demand a share of the savings, as providers assume the responsibility for utilization management. HMOs accustomed to taking 20 percent of premium dollars may find that amount reduced to 10 to 13 percent as they are forced to share revenues with their provider networks.

FIVE MODELS FOR NETWORK OWNERSHIP AND ORGANIZATION

The market wants integrated delivery networks consisting of hospitals, physicians, and insurers and HMOs. There are five possibilities for who will organize and own the networks:

Network Model I. HMO or Insurer

Health maintenance organizations and insurers are moving to tighten their networks and exercise greater control over providers. Pennsylvania-based U.S. Healthcare does not typically contract with multihospital systems or hospital-sponsored physician-hospital organizations. As the largest HMO on the East Coast, U.S. Healthcare has created its own network of 20,000 doctors and more than 400 hospitals. In a three-year strategy for tightening control, U.S. Healthcare reduced the number of providers by 50 percent, shifting to multi-year agreements for hospitals and physicians that meet the HMO's criteria. U.S. Healthcare's merger with Aetna will place this aggressive HMO in position to control 11 million covered lives, increasing the HMO/insurer's market clout.

In New Jersey, the Blue Cross plan has engaged in Darwinian pruning of its provider network. The plan announced in 1993 that it was converting its 2 million members to managed care and would be channeling those enrollees to only 56 of the state's 85 hospitals (Cochrane 1993a). The move shrank the physician network by 30 percent, as 13,000 physicians were affected when their hospitals were dropped. A New Jersey Blue's spokesperson said: "Doctors have to realize they are not characters in a Norman Rockwell painting." Physicians and hospitals were outraged and moved immediately to respond. Nine hospitals sued Blue Cross, and the state legislature prevailed on the plan to continue five indemnity options, in addition to the HMO.

For real control, some insurers and HMOs are acquiring doctors. Large health plans like Aetna and Prudential are establishing insurer-owned physician clinics. The insurers are purchasing existing physician groups or recruiting doctors into salaried practice for the health plans. Prudential is aggressively moving into the Raleigh, North Carolina, marketplace. The insurer opened the first of a planned seven clinics in 1994 and has expanded the strategy into other states. With 3.7 million enrollees, the insurer has managed care programs in 48 cities (Cochrane 1993c). Creating its own medical care delivery system will help Prudential compete with staff-model plans like Kaiser (Hamer 1994). As of 1993 Prudential has managed care programs in 48 cities, and 3.7 million enrollees (Cochrane 1993c).

Network Model 2. Hospital or Health System

Hospitals and health systems are aligning themselves in regional delivery networks. In Omaha, Nebraska, Alegent Health, a physician-hospital organization, has partnered with the Mutual of Omaha Companies to provide the first fully integrated managed healthcare system in the area. The insurer uses the Alegent provider network for its Omaha-area HMO, ExclusiCare.

Members of group purchasing organizations like Voluntary Hospitals of America are logical sponsors for regional networks. In

Tennessee, nine VHA nonprofit hospitals affiliated with Voluntary Hospitals of America formed the Middle Tennessee Network to pursue joint business opportunities such as managed care contracting and HMO development (Sherer 1994). Six of the hospitals are government-sponsored. The network constitutes a "super-PHO" that is creating links with other regional medical centers to create a statewide network.

The largest integrated delivery networks will need to regionalize their management and strategies. Sutter Health System in Sacramento, California, owns and manages 14 hospitals from the Central Valley to the Oregon border (Cerne 1994). Sutter is creating three regional organizations to integrate more effectively its acute facilities, skilled nursing homes, physician care centers, freestanding diagnostic and treatment facilities, medical groups, and health plans. To build its physician base, Sutter has created medical foundations in each region, providing access to tax-exempt capital for physician offices and group practice acquisition. Sutter-owned Omni Health Plan, with 80,000 HMO enrollees, is a joint venture with the St. Joseph's Medical Center in Stockton. Sutter's integrated HMO and facilities network has cost it some business. Foundation Health, a Sacramento-based HMO with 180,000 covered lives in the region, is now building primary care centers statewide and moved its affiliation to Catholic Healthcare West, Sutter's leading competitor. Sutter's ultimate network may be statewide.

Network Model 3. Physician

Physician-dominated organizations that contract for large groups of managed care enrollees are of greater and greater importance. Capitated medical groups are contracting independently with HMOs and insurers. Doctor groups can assume global capitation risk for all health services, then subcapitate or subcontract with hospitals and other physicians. In Worcester, Massachusetts, the Fallon Clinic is the hub of a multiservice network of two hospitals, a multispecialty clinic, an ambulatory care network, and an HMO. Fallon is expanding its penetration of central Massachusetts.

Over time, other medical groups that would follow Fallon must build or buy a comprehensive service network until they have all services "under one roof" (Cochrane 1993a). For physician groups to succeed, they must develop the capital and the management infrastructure for growth. The physician equity model is drawing considerable attention from doctors and has a significant market advantage in recruiting physicians and growing by noncash mergers with other medical group practices. The ability of this model to build a primary care network will make it a strong force in managed care and health reform.

For an example of regional networks, the Bay Physicians Medical Group in northern California took the lead in creating a for-profit management service organization that served as the full-risk contracting agent for the physician group and Alta Bates Medical Center in Berkeley (Droste 1994). This super-IPA linked 835 physicians affiliated with three local independent practice associations. The organization held contracts for 65,000 covered lives. Equity stock is held fifty-fifty between physicians and the Alta Bates system. Doctors hold a majority vote on all operating decisions, with five physicians and three medical center representatives on the super-IPA board.

Network Model 4. Partnership

The goal of the HMO-provider partnership model is to combine the insurer or HMO's enrollees and managed care marketing expertise with the provider's facilities, caregivers, and cooperation for cost management (Coile 1995b). Partnership models share equity and governance to align incentives and reduce the internal costs of provider-versus-payer.

Forming a true partnership between hospitals, doctors, and HMOs and insurers—a triad—may be the most difficult balancing act of all, according to Ray Barton, president and CEO of the St. Joseph Health System in Albuquerque, New Mexico (Barton 1994). But if the partners collaborate, this model can be the one with the best payoff for all parties. The St. Joseph Health System created a triad-model partnership with its physicians and FHP, a California-based health maintenance organization. St. Joseph owns three acute care hospitals in the Albuquerque metropolitan area. With its medical staff, St. Joseph has created Med-Net, a physician organization with more than 300 doctors, for managed care contracting under capitation. FHP has entered into a five-year contract with St. Joseph and Med-Net as exclusive providers for FHP's 35,000 enrollees. FHP patients account for more than 25 percent of St. Joseph's revenues. The triad partners cooperate in risk- and profit-sharing. A statewide expansion of their partnership model may be the triad partners' next step.

As mentioned in Chapter 8, Blue Cross and Blue Shield in Cleveland, Ohio, announced a strategic partnership for the creation of an integrated delivery system (Rudd 1994). The two organizations jointly offer several new health insurance products that will position Meridia, the region's largest hospital system, at the center of a new "super-Blue" provider network. Meridia linked with Blue Cross to fight its biggest rival, the University Hospitals Health System. According to John Burry, chair and CEO of Blue Cross, the goal of this payer-provider joint venture was to "revolutionize healthcare delivery in Ohio by integrating the functions of hospital care, physician services and insurance coverage" (Bader 1996, 19).

This alliance was complicated by the buy-out of Blue Cross and Blue Shield of Ohio by Columbia/HCA in mid-1996. Opposition to the deal flared immediately, as the Ohio attorney general moved to block the transaction (Jaklevic 1996). Columbia/HCA offered to acquire Meridia, but was turned down. Cleveland is shaping up as a three-system market, with the third major network organized by the Cleveland Clinic in partnership with the Kaiser Health Plan. Payer-provider partnerships that manage their costs through cooperation, not competition, may be the ultimate winners in the coming battle between major integrated delivery systems.

Network Model 5. Employers

Large employers and business coalitions may be potent network organizers. Employers are gaining real market clout with their managed care plans:

- CalPERS (California Public Employees Retirement System) won rate cuts from about 20 HMOs, including Kaiser (Anders 1995).
- Only 37 percent of American workers covered by health insurance are enrolled in traditional indemnity plans (Rosenblatt 1995).
- Big employers saw their health costs rise only 2 percent in 1994, according to a study of firms with more than 500 workers (Rosenblatt 1995).
- Shifting employees into managed care plans helped U.S. employers hold health expenses to only 1.1 percent in 1994 (*Los Angeles Times* 1995).
- Minnesota state employees were given a whopping 25 percent price cut by Medica, a Minneapolis-based HMO, in another example of aggressive employer contracting (Sardinha 1995).

Employers will have to keep up the pressure if they hope to win deeper premium reductions. In California, the Pacific Employers Group and CalPERS, who negotiate for 1.5 million enrollees, are encountering price resistance from PacifiCare and FHP, two of the state's biggest HMOs (Marsh 1996). If HMOs try to raise prices, employer coalitions could turn to direct contracting or "steering" enrollees to selected provider networks. In Cleveland, employers formed the Cleveland Health Quality Choice program, and demanded that local hospitals establish comparable databases for costs and quality. Following the second round of hospital data, the employer coalition revised benefit plans and demanded that their insurers contract with more efficient providers (Taulbee 1994).

Some employers fear that partnerships of physicians, hospitals, and insurers could become too powerful, dominating local markets and exercising noncompetitive market power. (Findlay 1993). In Racine, Wisconsin, the merger of the town's only hospitals, St. Mary's and St. Luke's, has created a potential powerhouse. Now the hospitals have purchased the area's two largest physician group practices and have begun to negotiate their contracts. Local employers are "outraged" at the creation of a "virtual monopoly" in town. Employers may invite the Aurora Health Network, based in nearby Madison, to provide more competition for employee healthcare contracting.

Providers and their health plans should get used to being put under the spotlight. "As purchasers of healthcare, employers want to be able to pass this information along to their employees," says Bridget Simone, a consultant at the Pacific Business Group on Health (Sanders 1995). Employers have focused primarily on costs in their coalition contracting efforts, but quality is next. As employer health costs come down, raising quality will be the corporate purchaser's next priority. Employers will pressure HMOs and insurers to demonstrate clinical outcomes and enrollee satisfaction.

In California, a coalition of employers, HMOs, and physicians released a comparative assessment of 21 HMOs statewide (Sanders 1995). The report card compared HMOs in six areas, including childhood immunizations, cholesterol screening, breast cancer screening, cervical cancer screening, prenatal care, and diabetic retinal exams. Health plans were analyzed using data from the National Committee for Quality Assurance.

BLUES REPOSITION FOR MANAGED CARE, MERGE PLANS FOR MARKETSHARE

How will traditional insurers like Blue Cross plans reposition themselves as newer HMOs take marketshare from the Blues' indemnity and preferred provider organization products? Market analyst John Cochrane (1993b) predicts "mega-mergers" among the Blues plans, promoted by volatile market shifts to managed care and accelerated by state-level health reform legislation in states like Florida, Washington, and Massachusetts.

If the 47.6 million BC/BS enrollees today converted to HMOs, America's HMO enrollment would double. Mergers could cut the number of independent Blues plans from around 60 to 40 over the next few years. BC/BS executives fear that Medicare will only deal with large plans in the future. Some Blues plans are converting to for-profit status, including Indiana, New Jersey, and Ohio. New York's Empire Blue Cross announced plans to convert to for-profit status in late 1996, prompting consumer groups to protest whether the conversion plan fits the public good (Freudenheim 1996).

Mergers and managed care dominate the Blues' strategic plans for the 1990s:

Illinois, Iowa, South Dakota. Blues plans in the upper Midwest are consolidating rapidly. BC/BS plans in Illinois, Iowa, and South Dakota announced merger agreements in May 1993 to create a super-Blues plan with 3.6 million enrollees and $4.1 billion in revenues. Streamlined administration and paperless processing with ATM-type cards would save millions in overhead.

Kentucky, Indiana, Ohio. A merger of the Kentucky Blues organization and the Associated Group of Indianapolis has created a huge new HMO, the Southeastern Group, with almost 2.5 million enrollees. Another merger is now in the works between the Associated Group and Community Mutual, the Cincinnati Blues organization, which would create a multistate plan with 4.2 million members.

Colorado, Nevada, New Mexico. Only the opposition of the Colorado Division of Insurance has blocked the potential merger of the BC/BS plans in Colorado, Nevada, and New Mexico. The plans have already created a joint marketing and management company, Rocky Mountain HealthCare Corp., even without state approval.

Rhode Island, Massachusetts. These New England Blues plans agreed in 1990 to share members across state lines, after the Rhode Island–based Group Health Association was acquired by the Harvard Community Health Plan from Massachusetts.

Former BC/BS Association president Bernard Tresnowski predicts, "If all health insurers play by the new rules, there will not be a unique role for the Blues. Many plans will merge or go out of business, but the strongest will survive and emerge even stronger" (Cochrane 1993b). Hospitals and physicians who are currently part of Blues provider networks should anticipate their plans' strategies (see Fig. 10.3). Providers should calculate whether

Figure 10.3 Blues Race to Integration for Managed Care: A Ten-Step Process

Step 1. *Traditional Indemnity.* Price remaining indemnity plans very high, with 15 to 25 percent annual increases to drive buyers into more integrated plans; eliminate unmanaged indemnity product.

Step 2. *Managed Indemnity.* Shift buyers and enrollees who want more choice out of managed indemnity into point-of-service (POS) plans, with lower prices for POS; eliminate remaining indemnity products.

Step 3. *Preferred Provider Organization (PPO).* Convert providers from discounted payments to capitation; eliminate providers who want to keep fee-for-service or per diem payments; shift enrollees and buyers who want more choice into POS plans by eliminating the PPO option.

Step 4. *Administration/Intermediary Services.* Shift self-insured employers into capitated HMO networks; offer POS as an option at a higher price for employers who want more provider choice.

Step 5. *Point-of-Service Plans.* Reduce the hospital-physician network for POS plans to capitated providers; charge higher premiums for POS plans' flexibility for out-of-network coverage.

Step 6. *HMOs.* Buy or build HMO plans under the Blue Cross/Blue Shield logo; shrink the provider network to hospitals and physician groups that will take capitation; convert other plan-type enrollees to HMO with lower premiums; buy marketshare from other HMOs with lowball 3 to 5 percent annual increases.

Step 7. *Capitate Providers.* Select hospitals, health systems, and physician groups for capitation; require performance accounting from providers; reduce BC/BS utilization and quality management overhead for higher HMO profits.

Step 8. *Blues/Insurers Mergers.* Expand marketshare by creating multistate super-Blues plans; purchase other insurers and HMOs to reduce competition and expand enrollment base; consolidate administrative expenses for higher profits.

Step 9. *Purchase Providers.* Purchase hospitals and physicians to build fully integrated HMO delivery system; reduce services network to wholly owned providers; focus on reducing clinical costs for higher profits.

Step 10. *Consolidate Mega-Blues Plans.* Merge Blues plans from 40 to 8 to 12 on a regional multistate basis; consolidate administrative positions and functions for higher profits.

their local Blues organizations will drop them, make them an acquisition offer, or initiate a long-term partnership relationship in the transition toward HMO models.

ACADEMIC MEDICAL CENTERS PARTNER WITH INSURERS

The nation's academic medical centers are making deals with insurers in a variety of partnership models. Academic medical centers have the potential to be partners with insurers and HMOs in integrated delivery, with their large salaried group of physicians that provide the core of a multispecialty group practice. Partnerships are blooming; the Massachusetts Blues plan and Massachusetts General/Brigham and Women's Hospital have announced plans to develop a Medicare HMO, jointly operate four ambulatory health centers, and share an integrated information system (Miller 1995a).

But teaching medical centers need a family practice delivery network that can provide geographic access and primary care. The University of Chicago Medical Center created a joint venture with the Meyer Medical Group, a 42-physician primary care group with four locations. (Golembesky, Harrison, and Muller 1994). The Meyer Group manages 50,000 covered lives in capitated contracts. The University's faculty "tracks" were expanded from four to five, creating a "clinical associate" category to provide a membership option for practicing community physicians. The university–group practice joint venture expands the University's primary care network. The goal of the partnership is to contract for a targeted 400,000 enrollees. Managed care accounts for more than 50 percent of the university hospital's case mix.

Minnesota's world-famous Mayo Clinic has built a regional network of local hospitals and medical groups in a 120-mile circle including southern Minnesota, Wisconsin, and Iowa. Mayo acquired or affiliated with providers in Eau Claire, Wisconsin; Austin, Minnesota; and LaCrosse, Wisconsin. Mayo now believes in managed care: "To bid effectively for managed care contracts, one has to have the integration of services . . . one has to have the delivery system in place," cites Mayo regional practice executive Michael Sullivan (Miller 1995b).

New models are being created for alliances and business relationships between academic medical centers and insurers or HMOs.

Carveouts. Insurers and HMOs are subcontracting specialty services to academic medical centers for bundled prices and volume contracting. In Atlanta, the Emory Clinic was selected by Cigna as the exclusive provider of cardiology services for all 68,000 of Cigna's HMO and point-of-service plan enrollees (Townsend 1994).

Self-insured plan management. University hospitals and health systems are contracting with insurers to manage the Universities' self-insured health plans. Since 1993, the Emory University EmoryCare plan, covering 11,000 employees and dependents, has been administered by Prudential.

Hub-and-spoke networks. Academic medical centers are acting as the hubs of regional delivery systems, in exclusive partnerships with insurers. In central Massachusetts, the University of Massachusetts signed a ten-year deal with New Hampshire–based HealthSource, a New England HMO. HealthSource agreed to develop and market a variety of HMO and self-funded managed care programs for employers, while the University provided a network of physicians and three community hospitals. The University plans to expand the network with additional hospitals while meanwhile maintaining its business relations with 40 other insurers and HMOs.

LOOKING FORWARD: HMOs AND INSURERS WILL SWITCH SIDES, INTEGRATE WITH PROVIDERS

HMOs and health insurers will shift their roles from representing purchasers to managing risk-sharing provider networks that contract directly with large employers, business coalitions, and state Medicaid programs. The low-inflation market is keeping them from making money on the purchaser side. Increasing price competition and direct employer contracting are forcing insurers to slash administration and provider payments if they are to remain profitable. HMOs and insurers racked up big profits between 1989 and 1992, with double-digit price increases. But real price competition is emerging among HMOs and insurers. In 1995, HMO prices actually fell, and purchasers sought even deeper price cuts.

Employers are no longer willing to pay 5 to 10 percent annual increases for indemnity health plans when HMO premiums rise only 2 to 4 percent or less. HMO premiums may be $500 to $800 less per enrollee than traditional plans. There are casualties in these price wars. The Travelers dropped out of the bidding for CalPERS enrollees after 1994 and eventually sold its healthcare business to United Healthcare of Minnesota.

Traditional insurers are now crossing the lines from insurance to healthcare delivery. In Arkansas, in another model of insurer-provider collaboration, Little Rock–based Baptist Health System has a joint-venture HMO with Blue Cross called Health Advantage. Baptist and Blue Cross then acquired HMO Arkansas, combining to form a new plan with 47,000 enrollees, which will serve two-thirds of the state. Under the restructuring, Health Advantage is owned 50 percent by Blue Cross, 25 percent by Baptist, and 25 percent by physicians affiliated with the plan. Across town, St. Vincent Infirmary Medical Center responded by bringing in an out-of-town HMO, HealthSource of New Hampshire. The new plan, St. Vincent HealthSource, is licensed in most of 75 counties in Arkansas. St. Vincent has another HMO venture with Prudential, in which St. Vincent is also the exclusive provider.

More insurers are opening ambulatory clinics, building or buying primary care networks, and developing their own staff-model delivery organizations. Prudential in St. Louis hired 20 to 25 primary care physicians in the mid-1990s, hoping to bring the total to 100 physicians by 1999. Dr. Jack Davidson of Prudential, the St. Louis plan's president and CEO, believes that the staff model is "what primary care physicians are looking for—more control of their own destiny (Cochrane 1993c). Doctors can invest in the group practices to gain an equity position. Prudential is only recruiting primary care physicians from internal medicine, pediatrics, and family practice. The doctors are forming new group practices of 7 to 8 doctors at facilities that Prudential builds or buys in the St. Louis metropolitan area to serve its 100,000 enrollees. Growth is forecasted at 225,000 by 1998. Prudential has reduced costs 15 to 20 percent in the 15 cities where it already operates group models.

Payer-provider alliances are focusing on community benefit as well as increasing marketshare, in response to a rash of HMO-bashing articles in the media. In Buffalo, New York, a local HMO, Independent Health Association, is sponsoring a $300,000 mobile health van that will provide outreach care to the underserved in upstate New York (Appelby 1996). The HMO has entered a partnership with Mercy Health System of Western New York, and the two companies have established a set of ethical guidelines for managed care contracting, which includes addressing the needs of the underserved in the region.

The future of American healthcare is an HMO world. Hospitals and physicians should expect that HMOs will be their purchasers, partners, and competitors. Ideally, providers will hold equity positions in their own HMOs and become partners with other managed care plans. Otherwise, hospitals and their doctors will be at a significant market disadvantage—vendors or competitors to stronger insurers and HMOs.

STRATEGIC IMPLICATIONS FOR PROVIDERS, HMOs, AND SUPPLIERS

Providers

Providers are at the low end of the food chain of managed care. They must become partners with HMOs and insurers who hold the enrollees, because managed care plans control the flow of payments and resources to the entire health delivery system. Providers have two choices: (1) work with HMOs and insurers in joint ventures and managed care plans, or (2) build provider-sponsored HMOs. The third option, "rent their network" to HMOs and insurers, is not a sustainable strategy. In a market with 30 to 40 percent excess hospital capacity and 30 to 50 percent excess physician specialists, providers are commodities with no market leverage.

HMOs

Managed care plans have the same three choices, but the perspective is different: (1) joint venture with providers; (2) build or buy their own facilities and physician groups; or (3) "rent" doctors and hospitals at market prices, usually at a substantial discount. Why should HMOs choose the partnership option? Because HMOs will ultimately compete on the performance of their provider networks, and the health plans do not have enough money to buy every provider they need. Partnership strategies are cheaper and better. HMOs must have the active cooperation of providers in delivering quality and customer satisfaction. HMOs that treat providers like commodities should not expect favorable treatment by "surplus" physicians and hospitals.

Suppliers

Suppliers must take care not to get caught in the competition between providers and HMOs. Pursuing partnership strategies with both managed care plans and provider networks may put the supplier "in the middle" between its customers. For example, the drug cost management systems now employed by companies like Merck may drive away hospitals and doctors whose drug use is being controlled by Merck's subsidiary. Taking sides will only offend another class of customers.

SOURCES

Anders, G. "CalPERS Discloses Rate Cuts of 3.8% from Health Plans," *Wall Street Journal,* 16 February 1995, p. B6.

Appleby, C. 1996. "Managed Care's True Values." *Hospitals & Health Networks* 70 (13): 20–23.

Bader, B. 1996. "The 'Grand Experiment': The Meridia Health System/Blue Cross Joint Venture." *Health System Leader* 3 (1): 19–27.

Barton, R. 1994. *The Healthcare Market "Triad."* Albuquerque, NM: St. Joseph Healthcare System (unpublished).

Cerne, F. 1994. "Sutter Health: Innovative System Faces Up to Challenges on the Integration Speedway." *Hospitals & Health Networks* 68 (21): 56–57.

Cochrane, J. 1993a. "The Ultimate Model for Integrated Healthcare?" *Integrated Healthcare Report* 2 (10): 8–11.

———. 1993b. "Can Health Insurers Survive?" *Integrated Healthcare Report* 2 (10): 1–7.

———. 1993c. "News Front: Prudential Insurance Company Sets Up Clinics in St. Louis and 15 Other Markets." *Integrated Healthcare Report* 2 (10): 13.

Coile, Jr., R. C. 1995a. "Managed Care Outlook 1995–2000." *Health Trends* 7 (5): 1–8.

———. 1995b. "The Future of American Health Care in the 'Post-Reform' Era." *Physician Executive* 21 (1): 3–6

Droste, T. 1994. "East Bay Medical Network: A Contracting Entity for Physicians and Hospitals." *Medical Staff Strategy Report* 3 (7): 2–4.

Findlay, S. 1993. "How New Alliances Are Changing Health Care." *Business and Health* 11 (12): 28–34.

Freudenheim, M. "Empire Blue Cross Is Asking New York State to Become a Nonprofit Company," *New York Times*, 26 September 1996, p. C6.

Golembesky, H., S. Harrison, and S. Muller. 1994. "University Medical Center Forms MSO with Private Physician Group." *Group on Faculty Practice Notes* 6 (4): 19–23.

Hamer, R. 1994. "HMO Industry Report." *InterStudy Competitive Edge* 4 (1): 1–109.

Jaklevic, M. 1996. "Ohio Attorney General Files Suit in Columbia/Blues Deal." *Modern Healthcare* 26 (29): 14.

Los Angeles Times. 1995. "Health Costs Fall with Big Push to Managed Care," 14 February 1995, pp. D1, D7.

Marsh. B. "HMO Premiums Are Heading for California Workers," *Los Angeles Times,* 30 July 1996, pp. D1, D15.

Miller, J. 1995a. "Mass Blues and Mass General/Brigham Form Partnership." *Integrated Healthcare Report* 4 (12): 19–20.

———. 1995b. "Mayo Expands Growing Network." *Integrated Healthcare Report* 4 (12): 14.

Palsbo, S. E. 1994. "1993 HMO Market Position Report." Cited in *Medical Benefits* 11 (1): 1–2.

Rosenblatt, R. A. "HMO Bandwagon Rolls On, But Not All Are on Board," *Los Angeles Times*, 21 February 1995, pp. D1, D3.

Rudd, T. 1994. "Ohio Blues and Hospital Network Confront Cleveland Rivals with an IDS." *Healthcare Systems Strategy Report* 11 (15): 12.

Sanders, E. "HMO Checkup: Study Rates Quality of Care Given in State," *Los Angeles Daily News*, 23 February 1995, p. B1.

Sardinha, C. 1994. "Competition, Employer Clout Push HMO Premiums Down 1.2%." *Managed Care Outlook* 7 (24): 5.

———. 1995. "Price Cuts Help Medica Win Market Share and Improve Risk Selection." *Managed Care Outlook* 8 (2): 1–2.

Sherer, J. 1994. "Central Tennessee: Not-for-Profits Band Together to Compete." *Hospitals & Health Networks* 68 (13): 50–51.

Taulbee, P. 1994. "Cleveland Firms Form Provider Panels Using Outcomes Data." *Managed Care Outlook* 7 (1): 6–7.

Townsend, R. W. 1994. "The Emory System of Health Care." *Group on Faculty Practice Notes* 6 (4) 1–5.

CHAPTER 11

Governing the IDN: New Models for a Post-Reform Environment

In the long run, the community care network will be the focal point of health care governance. And that's an area where we have the least knowledge, the least experience, the least preparation and the least capability.

Lawrence Prybill, Daughters of Charity National Health System
(Orlikoff and Prybill 1994, 60)

FUTURE HEALTH systems will be integrated delivery networks of cooperating hospitals, physicians and other caregivers, and health plans or HMOs. IDNs should not be confused with multihospital systems. Healthcare networks are loosely coupled organizations whose ever-changing partners are linked by contracts, not ownership. They are regional and statewide arrangements of providers and payers, contracting and assuming risk to provide a comprehensive scope of services to large enrolled populations.

All integrated delivery networks will engage in capitation, direct contracting, and risk assumption. Tough-minded networks must begin to consolidate services and settings. Is the U.S. healthcare system ready for such a jolting transformation? The post-reform environment will require leadership and radically new approaches to organization and governance.

Networks are a new competitor for multihospital systems. The nation's 250-plus multihospital systems are financially successful, piling up record profits in the 1990s (Greene and Lutz 1994).

But asset-merged systems are capital-intensive and slow to grow. Mergers can take two to three years to gain approvals, pass due-diligence analysis, and reconcile bond covenants. On the other hand, networks can be constructed quickly and cheaply in a matter of weeks, not years, by voluntary agreement among the participants.

Is a network a sustainable model? That remains to be seen. The concept is very new, with few models more than a few years in operation. Networks may be temporary, put together for a single purpose, such as an employer purchasing coalition or Medicaid contract. Insurer- and HMO-organized networks exist only on an annual basis, from contract to contract, with no guarantees of future participation.

Today's networks may turn out to be only a transition strategy, a trial marriage that will be followed by mergers. But networks may well prove to be more lasting institutions, a true organizational innovation of twentieth-century healthcare. If they continue to perform over time, networks may turn out to be durable, highly flexible delivery organizations.

GOVERNING THE NETWORK—WHATEVER IT IS

Networks will be governed under fundamentally different incentives than traditional hospitals or multi-institutional systems. Under capitation, the networks will be given incentives to reduce patient care costs, not to fill hospital beds or physician waiting rooms. Their customers will be enrollees, not patients. Networks will compete on the price of comprehensive packages of healthcare benefits and assume full financial risk for all services to their enrollees.

Unlike traditional multihospital systems, networks are more likely to be closing hospitals than expanding them. Experience in heavily capitated systems is that hospital utilization will decline by 35 to 50 percent, or more. But, given the incentives of capitation, empty hospital beds may be evidence of success, demonstrating that care management programs are working. This new mindset will call for entirely new models of governance.

Who owns a network? Everyone. Networks are joint business ventures that bring together hospitals, physicians, health plans and HMOs, and continuum-of-care providers. Many networks will be organized as stock companies or joint ventures. Ownership shares will vary, depending on capital investment. Those with the deepest pockets, including health plans and hospitals, will probably own a larger slice of the IDN pie. To ensure physician commitment, doctors are likely to be given a bigger share of governance and equity

(Bolinger 1994). Physicians can contribute capital by merging their practices and medical groups with the IDN or by paying for their investment stake with sweat equity and retained earnings.

Managing such loosely structured networks will be expensive in terms of communication and coordination. Linking the providers will require multimillion-dollar investments in community health information networks (Morrissey 1994). Physicians will need to be organized into regional primary care networks. The IDNs may purchase some physician practices. Specialists must develop systemwide protocols for cost-effective patient care. Many networks will start their own HMOs.

The challenge of governing tomorrow's IDN-model healthcare organizations is daunting. Unlike multihospital systems, networks may not own all their facilities or employ physicians. They will be in partnerships between hospitals, physicians, and health plans. This model relies on cooperation and collaboration. Network governance will be consensual, driven by a shared vision. The test of the network model will be managed care and capitation. Budgets will be tight. If network partners can manage utilization, control costs, and exercise self-discipline, they will succeed. Anything less than full cooperation will doom the network concept and perhaps the country's voluntary health system.

NEW GOVERNANCE MODELS FOR IDNs

Because networks are new, there are few successes—or failures—to provide models. Governance will be a hybrid of hospital boards, physician partnerships, and HMO corporate directorships. Key issues in structuring IDN boards are expertise, representation, and experience. All major stakeholders will be represented, including hospitals, physicians, and insurers and HMOs. The emerging array of IDN models is likely to take a variety of approaches to organizing governance and selecting directors:

Medical Clinic Model

Mayo, Cleveland, Geisinger, Fallon, Lahey, and Ochsner are medical clinic models. They are staff-model organizations, physician-governed and medically dominated. Medical clinic governance is by physician boards, although a few include up to 20 percent lay trustees. Most, if not all, directors of physician-led integrated delivery networks will be clinicians. Board meetings will be run like the executive committee of a hospital medical staff. Chiefs of major services will be board members, and clinical topics will be just as likely to get board attention as finance or market issues. Scientifically trained physician directors want data before making decisions. Governance decisions will be generally collegial, but service departments will be given deep discretion to manage their own budgets and clinical affairs.

Large medical clinics are organizing regional networks on the hub-and-spoke model, with the clinic as the nucleus of the delivery system. Regionally dominant clinics are the organizing centers of networks of community hospitals and physician group practices, built through affiliation and acquisition. Mayo, for example, has drawn a 120-mile circle around its home base in Rochester, Minnesota, and is acquiring local hospitals and smaller medical groups in the region. To compete in a world of managed care and capitation, the medical clinics must have decentralized primary care networks (Rodat 1994). Strategically minded medical groups are opening multisite primary care networks to serve a regional market.

Many medically sponsored IDNs will have their own HMOs. A growing number of the largest medical clinics, like Fallon, Geisinger, and Ochsner, are building successful HMOs to enroll patients and channel referrals to their clinics. Other medical clinics are engaging in HMO joint ventures, such as the one between Cleveland Clinic and Kaiser Permanente. They know that clinical prestige alone will not sustain a clinic. A regional network and HMO partnership are essential ingredients for the continued success of medical clinics.

Hub-and-Spoke

In the hub-and-spoke networks organized by academic medical centers and large regional hospitals, there is no question about who is in charge. It is the hub medical center, whose representatives dominate the board and select the network CEO. The balance of power in most decisions will favor the center. These will be heavyweight boards, whose decision makers will be deans, renowned physicians, corporate CEOs, and local elected officials. Real decision making is likely to be closely held in an executive committee controlled by the hub center.

Every metropolitan area that is home to an academic medical center is likely to have a hub-and-spoke network (Russell 1994), In Cleveland, Ohio, two dominant medical centers are giving local hospitals a choice of network affiliation. The Cleveland Clinic and University Medical Center are aggressively recruiting local facilities, acquiring physician groups, and lining up local health plans to provide the financing mechanism. Another powerhouse network has emerged in St. Louis, Missouri, where regional centers Barnes and Jewish linked with the Christian Health System. More than a dozen hospitals are in the Barnes-Jewish-Christian orbit.

Multicenter Network

Some regional healthcare organizations will deliberately choose not to have a dominant medical center. This could be called the string-of-pearls model, with no central hub facility. The founding hospitals may have strong tertiary centers of excellence, with costs that are 25 to 40 percent lower without the academic center's overhead. Well recognized in their own communities, these large hospitals do not want to play second fiddle to an academic medical center.

Competing regional hospitals may organize a multicenter network as a defensive strategy to counter the hub-and-spoke model. In Baltimore, for example, four local hospitals organized a multicenter network with no hub (Rudd 1994). They did not want the carrying costs of an academic center. Johns Hopkins is the centerpiece of a competing seven-facility network, with hospitals across greater Baltimore and suburban Washington.

Governing the multicenter network may be an excercise in diplomacy. Each medical center will have a block of trustees, according to how many beds or how much revenue each center brought to the table. Decision making is likely to involve elaborate behind-the-scenes arrangements between the major players, trading votes and influence.

Who will be strong enough to run multicenter networks? None of the hospital CEOs is likely to be acceptable to the others. Multicenter networks might better hire an executive with association experience. They may not tolerate a strong leader. In such a Byzantine political environment, CEOs could have short careers. These executives will need multi-year contracts and "parachute" payoffs in case they offend one center or another.

Public System

In large urban centers, public hospitals may form their own networks. The most important incentive may be Medicaid contracting. Some 20 states have been granted or have applied for waivers to permit managed care Medicaid contracting, and as of 1995 11.6 million Medicaid enrollees were in HMOs. Governing public hospital networks will be extremely political. Trustees will be political appointees. Hospitals will defend their own turf behind community advisory boards, and unions of public employees will fight to protect jobs.

Public networks could be very noisy to govern, with open competition between hospitals, medical staffs, union workers, neighborhoods, and City Hall. Unless they can overcome their infighting, public networks may struggle for survival against powerful medical center networks or HMOs that are competing for public patients.

New York's Health and Hospitals Corporation manages a network of public facilities across the five boroughs. The mayor has suggested turning over the management to a new company, even a for-profit contractor. The corporation is on the defensive now, competing for Medicaid HMO patients with emerging networks organized by leading medical centers like Cornell and Columbia-Presbyterian. Threatened cutbacks to Medicaid and Medicare could lead to $100-million fiscal shortfalls. The New York scenario demonstrates how public hospitals must not become isolated from other community-based networks.

Enterprise Model

Can for-profit corporations harness the incentives of enterprise to create a sustainable model? Wall Street is betting billions on companies like Columbia/HCA and Tenet. Proprietary hospital companies and HMOs can offer stock to provider partners. Columbia/HCA has experimented with offering physicians a chance to purchase ownership of up to 20 percent equity in local hospitals. Physician companies like PhyCor and Caremark/MedPartners are building physician networks through acquisition of medical group practices.

Governance in a for-profit setting will be strongly centralized in a corporate board of directors. Management influence will be high, with senior officials holding a third or more of board seats. For-profit hospital companies may put a doctor on the board to symbolize physician involvement. HMOs may add hospital or physician representatives. At the local level, regional network advisory boards of physicians and hospital executives will coordinate strategy and promote cooperation. But the regional networks ultimately do not hold the power. Real decision making in the enterprise model will be closely held by the corporation.

Provider-Payer Partnership

In this network model, the lambs lie down with the lions in a provider-payer partnership. The acquisition of the Graduate Health System in Philadephia by California-based FHP is an illustration of the provider-insurer trend. This tradition-breaking merger may succeed, where the proposed affiliation between California Blue Shield with UniHealth, a southern California hospital company, fell apart in 1993 over issues of corporate culture and leadership. Partnerships will not come easily, as provider-payer relations have become hostile in some markets. California providers have unsuccessfully attempted to enact legislation that would limit HMO administrative costs and profits to 15 percent of premium (Sardinha 1994).

Traditional adversaries will construct their governance structures carefully, before full trust can be gained through shared experience. There are likely to be supermajority provisions, which require that certain classes of decisions must be reached by a two-thirds or three-fourths majority of the board, and explicit protections against unilateral action by one party over another. Provider-insurer partnerships may be one-sided, where the insurer has acquired the delivery system, or vice versa, when the hospitals own the health plan. Board chairs and CEOs will be strong, highly respected individuals. They will have to be!

Making this partnership work may be complex and fractious, as providers and insurers attempt to blend their very different cultures. Provider-insurer mergers could have trouble with physician relationships. Doctors may fear the concentration of power between insurers and hospitals will leave the physicians out.

Seattle's consumer-owned HMO, the Group Health Cooperative of Puget Sound, strengthened its strategic position in an alliance with the Virginia Mason Medical Center and its regionally renowned Virginia Mason Clinic. Group Health serves 500,000 enrollees, in competition with the Sisters of Providence, a multihospital system with its own HMO and PPO, as well as a new hub-and-spoke network being organized by Swedish Medical Center. Physicians will be key members of these provider-insurer partnerships. Minnesota's Allina, for example, includes a fifty-fifty governing board of lay and physician representatives. To avoid conflict of interest, a number of the physician directors come from outside the region.

Community Partnership

An innovative set of community-led initiatives are developing a coalition approach to managing healthcare. In Orlando, Florida, the Disney organization created a new town, Celebration. A visionary design team conceptualized Celebration Health (Bezold, Corr, and Morrison 1994). The goal was a healthy community. This radically reoriented network begins with home settings, primary care nurses, and the information highway. Hospitals and acute care are last-resort resources. Florida's health reform program will ensure access for all Celebration residents. Providers expect to be capitated and to share risk for all health service needs.

Consensus and coalition building will be the governance strategies of community partnership networks. There will be no mistaking who is in charge. It is the community. Healthcare providers will hold minority stakeholder positions. Representatives of business, local government, civic organizations, and consumers will dominate the decision-making process. This is democracy in action, to create a community-based alternative to traditional provider-dominated health systems.

The community partnership network will set a broad action agenda, based on an assessment of community health needs and consumer expectations. Immunizations are likely to get higher priority than health facility improvements. Community partnerships will adopt report-card standards based on health status and consumer satisfaction. The community partnership model is the twenty-first century embodiment of a nineteenth-century concept—healthcare as a social institution, available and accessible to all, with a commitment to caring as well as curing.

CREDENTIALING THE IDN BOARD

Should $1-billion health systems be managed by amateurs, lay trustees with no expertise in healthcare management? Governance consultant James Orlikoff has concerns about the ability of health system boards to provide leadership for regional mega-systems (Orlikoff and Prybill 1994): "We don't have a strong base from which to get there; there's a tremendous degree of variance in terms of governance sophistication and definition of governance roles. Boards have gone through three or four levels of transition, and now we have to make a quantum leap to the next one."

Should there be *credentialing* of trustees and directors of integrated delivery networks? Future health networks may set very explicit criteria for serving on the board. One of the most important factors in selecting a board member may be prior governance experience. Evidence emerging from a long-range study of nine integrated systems suggests that the successful ones are governed by trustees who have already had experience at the institutional level, according to Stephen Shortell of Northwestern University (Sherer 1994). Experienced IDN directors may serve on multiple boards, as is common in the corporate world. Some Catholic healthcare systems actively share religious trustees on an intrasystem basis.

Well-managed integrated delivery networks may set criteria for their directors, including:

- health organization trusteeship (e.g., at least a 300-bed hospital or system with $50 million to $100 million combined revenues, or a 50-physician medical group practice);
- directorship experience of three years on the board of a large private-sector corporation or nonprofit organization;

- specific professional expertise (e.g., business, law, medicine, nursing);
- cosmopolitan outlook, not local provincialism; and
- demonstrated record of community service.

ALLINA HEALTH SYSTEM: A MODEL OF COOPERATION

Allina, the merger of Minnesota-based HealthSpan and Medica, is a model for the next level of evolution for integrated delivery networks. It brought together the dominant multihospital system and the second-largest HMO in the Twin Cities, linking healthcare financing and delivery for some 300,000 enrollees. This is a collaborative partnership, symbolized by coexecutives who jointly manage the new system.

Perhaps Allina could only have happened in the "cradle of managed care." More than 20 years ago, Paul Ellwood of InterStudy coined the phrase "health maintenance organization." Ellwood's HMO concepts rapidly gained favor from major employers such as Honeywell and General Foods, who converted their employees to HMOs. Providers responded by organizing multihospital systems like Fairview, Health Central, and HealthEast, and doctors clustered in group practices.

Today, Minnesota's health costs are among the lowest in the nation. Allina competes against other integrated delivery networks, including Health Partners, the region's largest staff-model HMO, and a new partnership between the Aspen Medical Group and Blue Cross, the Aspen Plus Health Network.

Gordon M. Sprenger, HealthSpan CEO and a past chair of the American Hospital Association, makes the case for integration: "If the separate self-interests of providers—mainly hospitals, physicians, and health plans—continue to fuel their adversarial relationships, we'll never be able to address the delivery system's serious problems" (Grayson 1994, 39). By merging a regional delivery system with an HMO, Allina could become an integrated service network, under Minnesota's health reform initiative.

SEATS AT THE BOARD TABLE: BASED ON CAPITAL OR COOPERATION?

Every integrated healthcare organization must face the capital issue. Conflicts over capital are almost guaranteed, due to the inequalities in capital available to hospitals, physicians, and HMOs. Should governance stakes—board seats and supermajority provisions—be based on capital investment? Or will the spirit of shared governance overcome the partners' differing abilities to contribute capital? There are several ways of resolving the dilemma this poses for governance:

Unequal investment and supermajority provisions. Minority investors can be protected by supermajority provisions, when the partners do not have the ability to share equally in capital investment. This often occurs when one partner, (e.g., a health system, HMO, or insurer) wants to hold a disproportional share of the board seats (e.g., 51 percent) and is willing to contribute more capital. Smaller partners (e.g., physicians and hospitals) may contribute a minority stake and take a lesser share of the seats, with the protection of supermajority provisions.

All partners are equal. One simple way to cut the governance pie in an integrated healthcare organization is to give all partners an equal share in governance, regardless of their level of capital investment, or even without investment. For example, an integrated organization representing a health system and physicians may decide to share governance fifty-fifty, with equal board seats, even though the health system may contribute all startup capital.

Equal startup investment. To maintain a level playing field, partners may agree to equal shares of initial investment, even when the capital resources of the partners may be very unequal. All parties may agree to contribute equally to the startup phase, anticipating that the new organization will use debt for growth and development over time.

Convert assets to capital stake. To create capital for partnerships, the new venture may purchase assets (e.g., physician practices, IPAs, PPOs, HMOs) and convert them to stock equity in the organization. This is most likely to be helpful to physicians, who may have limited free capital for investment but who want to be full partners.

Sweat equity and retained earnings. A partner who does not have the cash to invest fully in the venture at startup may use "sweat equity" on retained earnings as a strategy for building a capital stake. Another partner, or the venture, may lend that partner the share in the initial capitalization, relying on retained earnings to repay the loan.

Nonprofit IDNs (integrated delivery networks) must be sure to avoid issues of inurement and conflict of interest. The current guidelines from the Internal Revenue Service are clear that only 20 percent of a nonprofit IDN's board may be composed of physicians who will have a business self-interest in the new organization. To bring the board of an IDN up to fifty-fifty (physician-hospital), the network may add other physicians to the board who reside outside the market area. Allina adopted this strategy.

The clearest solution may be to divorce capital investment from governance. One or more partners may own a majority stake in the new organization, while other partners have no capital investment but are given seats at the board table in recognition of their political importance. These are matters for the attorneys, along with any antitrust concerns that may arise, as federal agencies and state attorney generals develop more specific guidelines affecting IDN formation and structure.

LOOKING FORWARD: GOVERNANCE BY COOPERATION—NOT COMPETITION

The formation and governance of integrated delivery networks are based on cooperation, an almost un-American concept. The nation's health system is fiercely competitive, a reflection of the traditional virtues of self-reliance and capitalism. In the post-reform era of limited resources, hospitals and healthcare organizations must shift to sustainable strategies. In a word, they must cooperate. Here are a set of methods and mechanisms for fostering collaboration in a network model:

- shared vision by network founders;
- co-equal representation of all participants;
- supermajority rules to protect smaller stakeholders;
- shared economic risks and rewards under capitation;
- commitment to eliminating redundancy in services and settings;
- coexecutives to share management responsibilities;
- protocols to manage clinical practice and reimbursement;
- vertical integration between services and settings;
- multifunctional teams;
- consolidation of support functions;
- networkwide focus on quality; and
- report cards on health status and consumer satisfaction. (Coile 1994)

Shared vision is first on this list because it is most important. Shared vision is what will transform traditional competitors—hospitals, physicians, insurers, and government regulators—into partners for community health. Each community-based vision will be unique. Everyone knows that resources will be limited, but even when all parties agree to "share the pain" of declining reimbursement, creating reallocation solutions that do not excessively punish one sector will be a real challenge for healthcare leadership.

Managed care and health reform are at hand. Ready or not, networks will be slammed together in the next few years (Kertesz and Wojcik 1994). Eventually, though, healthcare's game of musical chairs will be complete. Providers will have joined viable networks or they will be isolated and left behind. Governing network-model organizations will be a challenge. Win-win solutions will be hard to find. Overcoming turf issues and sharing capitation payments will require cooperation on a scale unprecedented in the health field. Somehow, it has to work. If network collaboration fails, the future is clear—a government-led takeover and the end of the voluntary health system in the United States.

STRATEGIC IMPLICATIONS FOR PROVIDERS, HMOs, AND SUPPLIERS

Providers

The integrated delivery network is a whole new ball game for providers, with new rules and roles. Hospitals will no longer dominate regional delivery systems. New models of shared governance will bring physicians into positions of control, at the IDN board level and as IDN executives. Nonphysician hospital administrators and trustees who are unwilling to share power with the clinicians in network management will find their best physicians escaping to competitors. Physicians cannot be held captive on hospital campuses. Doctors are likely to establish independent physician organizations and negotiate from strength with hospitals and HMOs.

HMOs

In the next few years, there will be a war between providers and HMOs and insurers in many markets over control of the IDNs. Health plans that try to dominate providers are destined to fail. There is no future for HMOs and insurers in perpetuating the tactics of discounted provider payments and micromanagement of provider performance. HMOs that are unwilling to capitate providers will create their own competition. Provider-sponsored HMOs are an entirely predictable response to the unwillingness of health plans to create real partnerships with providers.

Suppliers

The emergence of the integrated delivery network will create new customers—and new competitors—for suppliers. IDNs are very likely to create their own relationships with suppliers, bypassing existing group purchasing organizations like the Voluntary Hospitals of America and American Healthcare Systems. Statewide and multistate IDNs may create their own purchasing organizations and supply chains. IDNs will want deeper discounts, better service and support, and partnerships in product development. Product loyalty and compliance should be higher among IDN members than conventional GPOs, so IDNs may deserve preferred treatment from suppliers, manufacturers, and distributors. Large suppliers who ignore the IDN movement because of their established relationships with GPOs may find that IDNs have gone behind their back to cut preferred deals with smaller vendors and non-GPO products.

SOURCES

Bezold, C., C. T. Corr, and R. Morrison, 1994. "21st Century Health Systems: Principles and Visions." *Celebration Health and the International Health Futures Network*. Special Report. Institute for Alternative Futures. Alexandria, VA.

Bolinger, J. E. 1994. "A Guide to Developing Integrated Delivery Systems." *Medical Staff Strategy Report* 3 (6): 8–10.

Coile, Jr., R. C. 1994. "Managed Cooperation, Not Competition: A Proposal for Implementing National Health Reform." *Frontiers of Health Services Management* 10 (3): 3–28.

Grayson, M. 1994. "Sharing Power." *Hospitals & Health Networks* 68 (15): 38–43.

Greene, J., and S. Lutz. 1994. "Systems Post Fourth Straight Year of Income Growth." *Modern Healthcare* 24 (21): 36–49.

Kertesz, L., and J. Wojcik. 1994. "Risky PHO's Winning Bet." *Modern Healthcare* 24 (30): 44–48.

Morrissey, J. 1994. "The Future Starts Now for Regional Data Link-Ups." *Modern Healthcare* 24 (19): 52–60.

Orlikoff, J. E., and L. Prybill, L. 1994. "The Age of Denial: As Health Care Enters a New Era, Will Traditional Governance Survive." *Hospitals & Health Networks* 68 (15): 60–66.

Rodat, C. 1994. "Primary Care Development Strategies." *Health System Leader* 1 (2): 2–18.

Rudd, T. 1994. "Less Is More With Maryland's Newest Statewide Network." *Health Care Competition Report* 11 (12): 1–5.

Russell, B. 1994. "The Dynamics of Market Reform." *Integrated Healthcare Report* (April): 1–13.

Sardinha, C. 1994. "Plans 1, Doctors 0, in California Battle Over Profit, Cost Caps." *Managed Care Outlook* 7 (10): 7–8.

Sherer, J. 1994. "Merging Corporate Cultures: Turning 'Us' Into 'We.'" *Hospitals & Health Networks* 68 (9): 20–27.

CHAPTER 12

The Sixth Stage of Managed Care: New Models for the Post-Reform Era

A wave of mergers and alliances is transforming the nation's trillion-dollar health care system. Without waiting for the outcome of the Congressional health debate, providers of medical care—including hospitals, physician groups, and nursing homes—are joining to form bigger networks.

Milt Freudenheim (1994, A1)

AFTER THE healthcare system has been transformed by the five stages of managed care's rise to market dominance, after healthcare has been restructured into capitated networks, and after most Americans belong to an HMO, what comes next? Already, the innovators and leading-edge healthcare systems are looking for new trends and models.

There will, of course, be a sixth stage in the redevelopment of U.S. healthcare organizations. This final chapter of *The Five Stages of Managed Care* will speculate on what the next few years may bring.

TRANSFORMATION OF THE U.S. HEALTH SYSTEM IS AHEAD OF SCHEDULE

U.S. healthcare providers, payers, and purchasers are not waiting for Washington, D.C., to enact sweeping health reform. The transformation of the country's health system is already ahead of schedule.

Five Stages of Managed Care

HMO growth is accelerating, and capitation is spreading rapidly. Consolidation and networking among healthcare providers are rampant. The development of regional healthcare networks parallels the mergers among health insurers, HMOs, and industry suppliers. Most hospitals are joining networks (Freudenheim 1994). In 1994, the SMG Marketing Group of Chicago began to track integrated healthcare networks. By January 1995, SMG had identified a total of 291, involving almost 20 percent of U.S. hospitals (Henderson 1995). A year later, the number of networks soared to 504 (Henderson 1996). Many networks also own HMOs.

All parties are positioning themselves for the post-reform era when there will be 30 million to 40 million newly insured consumers. This could lead to a surge of demand—$50 to $100 billion in new healthcare expenditures. But that will not happen overnight. Health reform will be evolutionary, not revolutionary, phased in over years of progressive efforts to cover the uninsured, probably not until the federal budget deficit is back in balance, not likely before the year 2002. National health costs could balloon as occurred after the passage of Medicare and Medicaid in the 1960s, if the uninsured are suddenly given comprehensive health coverage with few controls on spending.

Tough marketplace contracting will reduce prices for services, and capitated providers will impose a new discipline on service demand. Large employers have been winning HMO rate rollbacks. Capitated medical groups and systems are lowering hospital use rates to unprecedented lows.

As employers and insurers dig in against rising expenditures, doctors are feeling the effect of market reforms, with pay cuts of 10 to 15 percent and more. The president of the Los Angeles County Medical Association says that in southern California, "Specialists like cardiologists, endocrinologists and neurologists are hurting, and very close to driving taxi cabs" (Greenberg 1994, B1). This is a national trend. Median pay for cardiologists dropped from $499,401 in 1992 to $446,990 in 1993, while radiologists went from $271,723 to $257,414, according to the American Medical Association (Greenberg 1994).

TEN NEW MODELS FOR THE SIXTH STAGE OF MANAGED CARE

What healthcare needs are new strategies and structures for reforming the U.S. delivery system. Advanced models are emerging from across the nation, especially in markets with high levels of

HMO and managed care penetration. Ten models may provide templates for re-envisioning tomorrow's systems:

Model 1. Consumer-Owned HMO

It is surprising there are not more consumer-owned health plans. The "mutual association" was a common early form of life insurance company, in which the policyholders owned the company and reinvested their dividends in it to increase growth. In the consumer-owned HMO model, thousands of consumers make up the investors who capitalize and manage their own health plan. A consumer-owned plan would put a high priority on customer service and on promoting the health of enrollees—the owners.

The most prominent consumer-sponsored health plan in the United States is the Group Health Cooperative of Puget Sound. This nonprofit HMO has enrolled more than 500,000 consumers in the Seattle area and is expanding across the Northwest. Consumers dominate its governance. Physicians are salaried, and most services are provided in facilities owned by Group Health. Its modern ambulatory clinics are strategically located to serve Group Health members. Group Health is a disciplined HMO with low costs and competitive premiums. Prescription drug costs are reported to be 28 percent lower than for a typical medical group (Group Health Cooperative 1993). Its market appeal has been based on benefit packages that are more comprehensive than those of competitors, and a reputation that it was run "for consumers." For example, Group Health offers premium rebates of up to 15 percent for consumers who practice healthy behaviors in seven risk areas, such as using seatbelts, exercising, and not smoking.

To strengthen its market position as one of the three dominant health systems in the Seattle area, Group Health negotiated a major strategic alliance with the Virginia Mason Clinic and Hospital, another staff-model organization. This should be a win-win partnership that brings Virginia Mason's clinical prestige and tertiary capacity together with Group Health's consumer base of a half-million covered lives. Group Health and Kaiser/Oregon announced plans to move into a closer market relationship, potentially creating a powerhouse nonprofit HMO in the Northwest.

Model 2. Statewide Network

A major market opportunity is emerging for providers to create statewide networks of hospitals and physicians. Hospitals in California, Oklahoma, and Texas are moving rapidly to do this. Some networks will be multistate. In the Washington, D.C., region,

Five Stages of Managed Care

providers are organizing to serve two states and the District. Greater Southeast and the Medlantic HealthCare Group are pursuing integrated delivery strategies for a region that will stretch more than 150 miles across Virginia to Maryland's Chesapeake Bay (Sandrick 1994).

In California, health systems are creating a statewide organization designed to pursue managed care contracting with large purchasers. Called the California Health Network, the partners include Sharp HealthCare in San Diego, Adventist Health System/West and Loma Linda University Medical Center in the Los Angeles market, California Healthcare Systems in San Francisco, and Sutter Health of Sacramento. The network will combine some 24 hospitals, 15,000 physicians, and 1.2 million managed care enrollees (Lafuente 1994).

The prime market opportunity for many statewide networks is Medicaid capitation contracts. Dozens of states are actively moving toward putting contracts out to bid for hundreds of thousands of Medicaid recipients. This is a big market. On a national basis, there are over 30 million Medicaid recipients. Those numbers could eventually grow if national health reform enfranchises the country's uninsured and Congress gives state governments the responsibility for getting them a health plan. This could mean that 15 to 20 percent of a state's population might be contracted out by state Medicaid agencies in the next several years.

California, Michigan, and Tennessee have already initiated Medicaid contracting, and more states will do so. By 1996, 13 states had received federal approvals to experiment with Medicaid reform. Some two dozen states have joined the Reforming States Group, which has been brainstorming solutions to problems (*New York Times* 1994).

Model 3. Brand Name Chain

Sears. K-Mart. Columbia/HCA. The concept of a national brand name works in every other sector of the economy. Why not healthcare? There will be brand name healthcare systems across the country. For-profit companies are working hard to create brand name chains of hospitals and regional networks (Lumsden and Haglund 1994). Columbia/HCA executive Richard Scott has appeared in his own television commercials. Surrounded by green-smocked workers, Scott pledged to reduce medical costs "not a little, but a lot" (Olmos 1995).

Columbia/HCA is the company off to the best start in establishing a national branded organization. With nearly 350 hospitals across the nation, it is aggressively targeting regional markets like Orlando, Florida, where the national giant acquired a 50 percent managing interest in 339-bed Winter Park Memorial Hospital, as the capstone of a four-hospital system (Lumsdon and Haglund 1994). Columbia/HCA is now in position to compete with networks owned by Florida Hospital and the Orlando Regional Medical Center. Columbia/HCA's acquisition of Medical Care America is paying off in Orlando, where the Dallas-based company operates seven ambulatory surgery centers. Medical Care America operates outpatient centers in 60 percent of the markets in which Columbia/HCA has hospitals. If Columbia/HCA is to be successful, it may need to purchase more hospitals. It may even purchase whole networks. Its three hospitals in the Chicago area are clearly not enough to make the company a real player in the sprawling 100-facility market.

In mid-October 1994, Wall Street was buzzing with rumors that a second 200-hospital mega-company could be in the making. Stories linking HealthTrust, American Medical Holdings, and National Medical Enterprises anticipated further consolidation among for-profit hospital management firms. HealthTrust, the former spinoff of Hospital Corporation of America, operates hospitals in a number of rural markets in which their facilities are often sole providers. HealthTrust's merger with Epic brought three continuum-of-care companies in home care, geriatric psychiatry, rehabilitation, and subacute care. HealthTrust ultimately chose Columbia/HCA, creating the nation's largest chain. Another for-profit chain has been active in healthcare: In March 1995, National Medical Enterprises and American Medical International merged to form Tenet Healthcare Corporation. Based in Santa Barbara, California, this 75-hospital chain had more than $5.5 billion in net operating revenues in fiscal 1996 and is emerging as a strong competitor to Columbia/HCA (Lutz and Gee 1995). Some brand name strategies are regional. OrNda, which merged with Summit, now operates more than a dozen hospitals in southern California. Stock prices are rising, as Wall Street bets that there will be national brand name chains in American healthcare.

Model 4. Provider-Payer Merger

True integration in healthcare requires a combination of financing and delivery. Staff-model HMOs like Kaiser and Group Health of Puget Sound can operate with as little as 5 to 8 percent administrative costs. The challenge for America's hospitals and HMOs is to find a common ground, merging to achieve real efficiencies in management while providing one-stop shopping for purchasers.

Insurer-provider mergers make increasing sense in a market-driven system, and the forces promoting integration will increase at each stage of managed care's market penetration. Key factors accelerating the integration of payers and providers include:

- price wars between HMOs and managed care plans;
- employer demands for reduced HMO administrative costs;
- HMOs' and insurers' need to cut patient care costs;
- employer coalitions' leverage to get HMO price cuts;
- purchasers' demand for data on provider quality;
- providers' surplus capacity needs for committed HMO volume; and
- capitation teaching providers how to manage costs.

In the long run, providers and HMOs will discover that it is less costly to cooperate than to compete. As employers demand lower costs and proof of quality, HMOs can reduce their costs by delegating to providers responsibility for managing patient care costs and quality. Why should HMOs and providers duplicate functions such as network management, provider credentialing, utilization management, and quality assurance? HMOs and insurers will learn that they are competing on the performance underlying provider networks. Staff-model HMOs with employed physicians have significantly lower administrative costs, in the range of 5 to 8 percent.

It may be easier for providers to start their own HMOs than to engage in the extensive due-diligence and organizational restructuring of a full merger with a managed care plan. InterStudy lists some 130 provider-sponsored HMOs in its national directory; they manage more than 10 percent of all HMO lives across the United States (Hamer 1996). Four successful models of provider-sponsored HMOs include:

Presbyterian Health Plan (Albuquerque, New Mexico). Presbyterian's current HMO is its second. The first was closed after physician dissatisfaction about HMO payments. The second HMO has 80,000 enrollees, and the system contracts for another 50,000 capitated lives.

First Option (New Jersey). Owned fifty-fifty by a network of 50 hospitals and 9,400 physicians, First Option is a true provider partnership. The hospitals contributed their employees to jump-start initial enrollment and turned a profit in only 14 months.

The plan covers 225,000 members and is competing hard with Aetna/U.S. Healthcare and Blue Cross for statewide marketshare.

General Health System (Baton Rouge, Louisiana). This health system's HMO, Gulf South Health Plans, has captured 32 percent of the market, with 60,000 full-risk lives and 150,000 enrollees. The HMO's growth has not been without tensions, as Gulf South has had to cut physician reimbursement to keep rates competitive.

Secure Care (Des Moines, Iowa). Mercy Medical Center launched its HMO cooperatively with its 320-physician medical staff and quickly grew to 10,000 enrollees through 50 contracts. In the long term, Mercy hopes to link its HMO into a statewide model in collaboration with other physician-hospital organizations (Rovner 1996).

Model 5. Public-Private Partnership

Many of the nation's largest hospitals are publicly owned teaching medical centers. A new model of public-private partnership may give these government-owned hub hospitals a distributed network of for-profit hospitals. Columbia/HCA is offering a merger proposition to Arizona's Maricopa County that would bring the national chain into a business partnership with the county's public hospital. Struggling with a $60.6 million debt burden, Maricopa County could use a partner with deep pockets and management expertise. A potential deal could unite the public hospital with Columbia/HCA's two for-profit community hospitals in Phoenix.

As for-profit chains run out of other investor-owned facilities to acquire, they are turning to purchasing nonprofit hospitals. For example, Columbia/HCA purchased the Samaritan Health System and San Diego–based Sharp Healthcare, which could give the big chain the position of market leader in the influential California market (Olmos 1995).

Model 6. Information Network

Hospitals and health plans may organize networks linked by the information highway. InterMountain HealthCare utilizes an extensive regional information system to link its two dozen facilities across five Western states. Well over $100 million has been invested in its award-winning community health information network. Lutheran General's CEO Stephen Ummel believes no integrated delivery system can function without an information system framework (Bergman 1994). Detroit's Henry Ford System uses telemedicine linkages to bring specialty care to remote areas.

Integrated networks will compete on their performance. That means data, translated into useful information and available across a region or statewide delivery network. The survivors in the managed care marketplace will be the providers and HMOs that use data to create a sustained competitive advantage. CHINs will provide the architecture and linkages for:

- managing patients in real time, with data instantly available on costs and quality;
- reducing length of stay and expenses per case by closely following computerized clinical pathways and "care maps";
- eliminating high-cost variations in patterns of care by individual physicians; and
- public reporting of costs, clinical outcomes, and patient satisfaction to major employers.

Developing network CHINs won't be easy. A recent panel of experts identified a number of issues facing America's healthcare information network pioneers:

- integrating diverse platforms of hardware and software across a network;
- making clinical information systems universally available, easily accessible, and relevant to clinicians;
- handling security, privacy, and confidentiality concerns;
- maneuvering through multiple vendor issues;
- strengthening the role of the chief information officer;
- potentially huge investments to create the information system architecture; and
- applying managed care protocols across a decentralized provider network. (Bergman 1994)

Employers are demanding comparative data from HMOs and providers. Sophisticated companies and business coalitions are requiring their HMOs and insurers to report data using HEDIS. The system is quickly becoming the industry standard for healthcare data (Miller 1995b). HMOs must report data on use of preventive care, member satisfaction, healthcare costs and utilization rates, and the financial stability of the health plan.

Strong leadership will be needed to bring the CHINs together. New partnerships will link hospitals, universities, vendors and governments to capitalize on expertise and maximize investments in research and development. Chief information officers must work closely with health system CEOs to put the necessary information environment in place to link these diverse settings and services.

National health information networks are coming. Health-OnLine is the first national on-line information service targeted for the health industry. Denver-based Kaiser Associates, a consulting firm, joined with Healthcare Forum in San Francisco to pioneer an electronic communications and information network (Lutz 1994). Health-OnLine has reached 350 users and has signed up the Catholic Health Association to link its 600-hospital membership.

Model 7. Virtual System

The "virtual" integrated delivery system relies on contractual linkages and business cooperation to create an integrated health system. Like the virtual company, this model owns no assets. It is a strategic alliance between health plans and providers, who align their organizations to share capitation and market management. The virtual system is the opposite of an asset-merged model. One example is the linkage between the Legacy Health System in Portland and Blue Cross/Blue Shield of Oregon. The two organizations share interlocking boards and have launched a joint managed care product with three large physician groups to compete against staff-model Kaiser and the Sisters of Providence.

Futurist Jeff Goldsmith recommends taking an alternative path to integration (Goldsmith 1994). The virtual system is based on market-specific affiliations between providers and established health insurers or HMOs. The partnership is built on shared values and vision. The principal assets are information systems and cash, not bricks and mortar. These systems can use sophisticated mechanisms for evaluating practice patterns, selecting preferred providers, and experimenting with incentives such as capitation.

Providers need to learn from network-model HMOs like PacifiCare of Fountain Valley, California, Humana of Louisville, Kentucky, and United Healthcare of Minneapolis, Minnesota, which do not own hospitals or employ physicians. These companies enter into multi-year arrangements with selected physician groups, hospitals, and health systems. Using contracts instead of capital, the health plans can move rapidly into a market, establish a provider network, and market themselves to local employers trading upon the reputation and capacity of the providers.

The secret to successful virtual integration efforts is a true partnership. In Albuquerque, New Mexico, the St. Joseph Health System has a five-year strategic alliance with FHP, a California-based HMO. The FHP agreement uses St. Joseph facilities and doctors on an exclusive basis. A senior administrator from FHP manages St. Joseph's hospitals. FHP is now more than 25 percent of St. Joseph's business, and growing. Creating a strategic alliance with St. Joseph has given local credibility to the out-of-state FHP plan. Both FHP and St. Joseph believe their strategic alliance is essential to compete with other local integrated systems, including the Lovelace Clinic, a staff-model clinic owned by Cigna, and Presbyterian, a statewide hub-and-spoke model with its own HMO.

Model 8. Physician Clinic

Physician-sponsored group practice "clinics," which integrate doctors, hospitals, and health plans, represent a sustainable model for tomorrow's health system. The nation's largest medical clinics are positioning themselves as integrated healthcare systems with a financing mechanism. James Unland of the Health Capital Group in Chicago believes physician-led networks will have an inside edge in future competition: "Physician-directed managed care organizations will become increasingly prevalent.... Physicians, particularly primary care physicians, will govern resource utilization in the future" (Unland 1994). He predicts that 70 percent of physicians will practice in groups of 10 or more by the year 2000.

The most successful clinics in the future will own an HMO. Larger clinics will own hospitals, although enlightened physicians will view hospitals as a costly expense center to be used as a last resort. In Danville, Pennsylvania, the Geisinger Foundation operates a multispecialty group practice, a hospital, satellite ambulatory facilities and a 160,000-member HMO. Geisinger's expansion under its nonprofit umbrella has been frustrated by opposition from the Internal Revenue Service, which has challenged Geisinger's bid to obtain 501(c)(3) status for its HMO (Burda 1994b).

Brand name medical groups will put their labels on HMO products. Prestigious medical groups may lend their brand name status to HMOs in return for a share in an HMO venture with insurers. Partnerships and joint ventures offer a low-risk way for big medical groups to get into managed care, with little or no capital contribution by the doctors. In Arizona, the Mayo Clinic announced a managed care partnership with national insurer John Alden Life Insurance (Miller 1995c). The partnership of Mayo Healthcare Network with John Alden in Phoenix will jointly market a new insurance product, with Mayo's 150 Scottsdale-based physicians as the provider network.

Model 9. Wellness Plan

The HMO concept is just now beginning to fulfill the implicit promise of "health maintenance." In California, the giant Kaiser health plan, is now aggressively identifying high-risk enrollees for targeted health promotion. As capitation gains market acceptance, more provider networks and health plans will increase their health promotion investments. Aetna's Philip Nathanson predicts that, on a long-term basis, promoting health will lead to improved financial performance: "We know, for instance, that every dollar we spend on pediatric immunizations saves $3 in costs down the road" (McManis 1994).

Progressive health systems are investing in community health. In New York's South Bronx, the huge 1,700-unit Melrose Commons housing project is being renovated to include health centers for the resident's impoverished population. New York's Department of Health and Hospitals is now renovating its network of 25 community health clinics like the Charles R. Drew Center, a satellite center of the Queens Hospital Center.

Health education is receiving a boost in New Albany, Ohio, from the U.S. Health Corp. The town is the site of a growing model community that will promote health awareness and lifelong learning. With assistance from U.S. Health Corp., a "healthy living" curriculum will be a model for education in grades 1 through 12. Students will keep journals and computer databases of their health status. A 2,000-square-foot Wellness Center is being constructed, adjacent to a senior center, to include health education, day care, health fairs, counseling, and examination and treatment facilities. Physicians from Riverside Methodist will provide backup services.

Model 10. Mega-Network

Network organizers are thinking big, bigger, and biggest. In Kansas City, Health Midwest merged with Menorah to create a 10-hospital system with 1,800 beds (Scott 1994). Two more facilities are expected to join the system. Today, most of the region's hospitals belong to systems or networks. Mid-America Health First operates 8 hospitals, and 5 hospitals have aligned with the 464-bed University of Kansas Medical Center in the Jayhawk Alliance, a hub-and-spoke model. The pot is bubbling in this market. Columbia/HCA has acquired two hospitals in the region, and Kaiser is planning to expand its HMO enrollment there through an alliance with one of the three mega-networks.

In Arizona, a linkage between Samaritan Health System and HealthPartners of Southern Arizona would create Integra Health System, the state's largest nonprofit health system (Lutz 1996). The deal could be expanded to include Mercy Healthcare of Phoenix, forming a system with nearly 3,000 beds. Next, Samaritan is weighing the potential advantages of a strategic alliance with a for-profit partner, such as Columbia/HCA, Tenet Healthcare, or OrNda. Nashville-based OrNda is the largest for-profit chain in Arizona, with six facilities, five located in Phoenix.

Another mega-network is shaping up in Dallas. Texas providers always think big. This time three of the largest nonprofit systems in the region are forming strategic business relationships, aligning Baylor Health Care System, Presbyterian Healthcare System, and Methodist Hospitals of Dallas. Mega-networks may dominate smaller markets, too. Roper Hospital and Bon Secours–St. Francis Xavier, in Charleston, South Carolina, discussed a merger, ultimately uncompleted, that would have combined 41 percent of the region's hopital beds in a three-facility organization (Burda 1994a). The construction of a mega-network must overcome local rivalries, including a bitter certificate-of-need battle over which hospital will build in a growing suburban sector.

Physician organizations—not hospitals—may be the building blocks for mega-networks. The Florida Independent Physicians Association, a statewide physician contracting network with 5,000 doctors in 11 regional organizations, covers all 65 counties in Florida (Miller 1995a). Now the sprawling medical network is creating a sixty-forty joint venture with the Coastal Healthcare Group of Durham, North Carolina. Coastal Healthcare owns HMOs and manages physician groups, combining the two businesses in such ventures as Doctors Health Plan, an IPA-model HMO launched in early 1995 to cover 27 counties of North Carolina.

The deals keep coming in diverse markets across the country, as the level of managed care penetration rises. In Cleveland, a Stage 3 market with 8 HMOs, the Cleveland Clinic and 8 other local healthcare organizations formed the Cleveland Health Network. To cover the northeastern Ohio market, Cleveland-area providers are aligning their market strategy for joint managed care contracting. They will compete with the Meridia Health System/Blue Cross venture, which anchors a 21-hospital regional network organized by the Blues (Bader 1996).

THE MOST INTEGRATED HEALTHCARE MARKET IN AMERICA

Anyone wanting a glimpse of a post-reform market should watch Minneapolis–St. Paul. If all U.S. hospitals were located in the Twin Cities, utilization would be 20 percent lower, saving the country an estimated $12 billion annually, according to Baltimore-based HCIA, a market research firm (Melville 1994). According to the researchers, 20 percent of hospital days would be rated "clinically unwarranted" if the Minneapolis–St. Paul Market were used as the standard.

Market-driven health reform started in Minnesota. This progressive state enacted health reform in 1992, with a target date of July 1994 for implementation, since extended to 1997. The plan for MinnesotaCare would pool Medicaid patients and the uninsured, and contract for care with local provider-insurer organizations called integrated service networks. ISNs replace HMOs and insurance plans, providing comprehensive care packages defined by the state. A mandate requires all employers to contract with ISNs for their employees. Fee-for-service will be an option, but hospital and physician prices will be regulated by the state. All hospitals and physicians must belong to at least one ISN. Consumers would have a choice of networks.

Legislative support for such a radical plan is waning now, but the result has been to encourage rapid integration among Minnesota providers and insurers and HMOs. There seem to be at least monthly mergers among hospitals, doctors, and insurers and HMOs in the Twin Cities. Developments include:

HealthPartners, the largest staff-model HMO in Minneapolis–St. Paul, formerly "rented" beds from several health systems. Now the HMO has added two hospitals to its base of 500 employed physicians, one facility on each side of the metropolitan area. St. Paul–Ramsey, the former public hospital in downtown St. Paul, has affiliated with the HealthPartners system, bringing with it a 200-physician clinic. The Park Nicollet Medical Clinic and Methodist Hospital in the west metropolitan area signed a ten-year agreement with HealthPartners. HealthPartners has been contracting with the Large Employer Initiative; it won the bid in 1992 to provide comprehensive healthcare to 150,000 enrollees from the biggest companies in the Twin Cities, but that contract expired at the end of 1996.

Blue Cross/Blue Shield of Minnesota is building a provider network through acquisitions and exclusive contracts. In 1994, Blue Cross completed the acquisition of the Aspen Medical Group, a 100-physician group practice with an excellent record in managed care. More physician practices, which Aspen will manage, are likely to be acquired. To provide hospital services, Blue Cross is contracting with the University of Minnesota hospital, allaying fears that the university might be excluded from integrated service network participation.

HealthSpan, a multihospital organization created in 1992 by the merger of the HealthOne and LifeSpan systems, is moving to reposition itself as an ISN serving the entire Twin Cities metropolitan region. HealthSpan is acquiring physicians and groups to solidify its physician base and has merged with Medica, the second-largest HMO in the area. Medica is a subsidiary of United Healthcare, one of the nation's largest HMOs. The new company, Allina, has coexecutives to oversee its managed care and delivery network divisions.

HealthEast, a system that once boasted nine acute hospitals in St. Paul, is moving strategically to create a fully integrated model that brings together the "above-the-line" insurer-HMO functions of marketing and finance with the "below-the-line" provider-delivered activities of patient care, quality assurance, and utilization management. HealthEast conducted an intensive "Constitutional Convention" planning process with key physicians and trustees. The result is a multitrack model with options for physician affiliation and ownership, potentially including a new for-profit holding company with equity shared by physicians. HealthEast is committed to a physician-friendly strategy of fifty-fifty sharing of governance and capital investment with doctors. The new model is driving reductions in hospitals and beds. In 1994, HealthEast cut back to three facilities. The system announced the closure of Divine Redeemer Hospital, converting the facility to long-term care and adding an ambulatory care center. In mid-1996, HealthEast announced plans to close Midway Hospital and open a small, 70-bed facility in the suburbs for better geographic distribution.

Fairview Health System, with six hospitals in the west metropolitan area of Minneapolis and suburbs has been building a primary care network through acquisitions and affiliations with doctors across its local market. Fairview CEO Rick Norling comes from California and has strong managed care experience. Fairview created a closed-panel physician-hospital organization that demanded exclusivity. Fairview doctors joining the PHO were prohibited from also affiliating with the physician network of Fairview rival HealthSpan. Fairview has been in discussions to strengthen its future with an alliance with Blue Cross, and has negotiated a merger with the University that will stabilize the future of the medical school.

HealthEast and *Fairview* with *North Memorial*, the last independent hospital in the Twin Cities, together held the small-employer coalition contract for three years to serve 200,000 enrollees of small and midsized employers. Prudential was the insurance partner but decided to exit the competitive Twin Cities market at the end of the contract. That opened the door to Medica, the region's second-largest HMO and newly merged with HealthSpan to form Allina, to win a five-year contract with the Minnesota Employers Association. Medica won another employer contract by offering Minnesota state employees a whopping 25 percent price reduction (Sardinha 1995). Now each has organized a local care system to participate in the direct contracting program with the large-employer coalition, beginning January 1997.

Rural Minnesota may also be a bellwether market for managed care trends in nonmetropolitan areas. Minnesota's Blue Cross/Blue Shield plan is moving to dominate out-of-state markets, with a series of provider partnerships around the state (Cochrane 1993). In southwestern Minnesota, the plan negotiated an arrangement with Affiliated Medical Center, a large rural group practice. A profile of Blue Cross data showed the doctors to have good cost profiles and lengths of hospital stays. Although the group had little managed care experience, it agreed to cover 14 counties in southwestern Minnesota. Blue Cross provided the information system and administrative support to the physicians. The Dakota Clinic, a 160-physician group in Fargo, North Dakota, will cover the northwest portion of Minnesota. The Minnesota Blues plan is positioning itself for certification as a statewide ISN.

STAGE 6 MEANS HOSPITALS SHOULD PREPARE FOR 0.8 BEDS PER 1,000

As the nation moves through Stage 3 and higher up the scale of healthcare transformation, many hospital boards and medical staffs still struggle with the effects of managed care and locally driven reform. The central purpose of tomorrow's healthcare organizations is to provide comprehensive health services to an enrolled population. Keeping hospital beds full is based on the old paradigm of fee-for-service reimbursement. Keeping enrollees healthy and out of the hospital is the new paradigm, which will propel the business, clinical, social, and moral mission of the healthcare organization in the future. Richard McCann, chair of the board of the Northeast Ohio Community Health Plan, advises, "The goal is not to fill the hospitals; it's to gain managed care business" (Bader 1996, 19).

From 1950 through 1980, the widely applied planning formula was "4 beds per 1,000." Government programs like Hill-Burton subsidized hospital construction across the country, using such bed-based formulas to grant millions of dollars in loans and guarantees, which led in time to the current surpluses of hospital beds. Compare that formula today with the performance of Mullikin

Medical Centers of Long Beach, California, which manages more than 300,000 HMO enrollees with an effective bed demand of 0.8 to 1.0 beds per 1,000. Most healthcare markets in the United States are substantially overbedded, with between 3.0 and 4.0 beds per 1,000 population. The California Healthcare Association's environmental forecast for the years 2000 to 2005 assumes that hospital bed demand could fall to as low as 0.6 to 0.8 beds per 1,000 in the twenty-first century (Coile and Menkin 1996).

There is evidence that the declining demand for inpatient care could bottom out at some level. HCIA, a healthcare research company, found that hospital stays rose slightly in 1995, to 5.1 average days, up from 5.0 days in 1994 (Anders 1996). HCIA analysts speculated that so many lower-intensity cases had been switched to ambulatory settings, that higher-acuity patients were driving up stays. Even with a stabilizing of length of stay, however, the problem of excess hospital capacity remains extreme. A downsizing of the hospital system is the inevitable next step in the transformation to a managed care marketplace.

LESSONS FROM OTHER INDUSTRIES FOR A VIEW OF THE FUTURE

Hospitals and physicians seldom look to other industries for inspiration in developing new models. This insulated attitude could be a mistake. For example, U.S. industry's experience with reengineering the corporation has lessons for hospitals. Futurists Ian Morrison and Greg Schmid, the authors of *Future Tense*, caution that adopting the reengineering approach in the health industry could be shortsighted. In other industries, downsizing has undermined consumer confidence and worker loyalty. Companies that leveraged core competencies by contracting out key functions weakened their ability to develop new products and services (Morrison and Schmid 1994).

Morrison and Schmid do criticize healthcare's "fractured" system of paying for care on an episodic basis. They predict that new organizations such as the Friendy Hills Health Care Network in southern California, with 200 primary care physicians and specialists and its own hospital, will be the integrating force that reinvents healthcare delivery. The Friendly Hills network is one of the most efficient capitation managers in the West, with utilization rates barely one-third of national averages. Acquired by Caremark, since merged with MedPartners/Mullikin of Birmingham, Alabama, the Friendly Hills network will now have the backing of a well-capitalized for-profit company for growth and expansion.

Stanford University Hospital engaged in a four-year reengineering program. In the process, Stanford looked at similarities between healthcare and airlines and banking (Sherer 1994). Stanford was searching for lessons from the experiences of these sectors. The airlines, for example, have been seeking solutions to the problems of overcapacity and variable demand. What can hospitals learn from Southwest Airlines' strategy of eliminating seat assignments and turning around their planes in less than 20 minutes at the gate? Business has a substantial experience in strategic alliances—the network strategy.

LOOKING FORWARD: THE PAST IS HISTORY. THE FUTURE IS NOW.

The era of a "kinder, gentler world" in healthcare is over. Now! Hospital administrators and physicians who believe they can pursue "transitional strategies" of maximizing revenues are doomed to failure. Halfway measures that hope to protect a freestanding, fee-for-service, go-it-alone world will not work in an integrated marketplace. Organizations that persist in clinging to the past are about to become history themselves, replaced with a new wave of healthcare and physician executives who will welcome capitation, and who will close hospitals without tears or a backward glance.

The new world of capitation and reform awaits:

- Healthcare delivery will be converted from a "retail" market to "wholesale" transactions for hundreds of thousands of enrollees.
- Price wars between HMOs, insurers, and self-insured provider networks will shake out smaller health insurers.
- Competition will drive the prices of health plans down to 3 to 5 percent annual increases.
- Providers will contract with a few, very large healthcare purchasers.
- Many health plans will acquire their own primary care physicians and use them as gatekeepers to hospital and specialty services.
- Hospitals and doctors will join one of three or four regional provider networks on an exclusive basis.
- Academic medical centers will become "niche" providers of a limited range of high-technology services.
- Demand for hospital beds will shrink by 15 to 25 percent in the next three to five years.

- Most—95 percent—of the 650,000 active physicians in the United States will join group practices or managed care networks within five years.

This is not the beginning of the end. It is the start of *twenty-first century healthcare*, a whole new era in providing community-based healthcare with a formula that emphasizes capitation, clinical protocols, ambulatory care, noninvasive surgery, and substantial reliance on alternative nonhospital settings such as subacute and home care. Healthcare can learn a lesson from other U.S. companies seeking to reinvent themselves: (1) create vision and leadership; (2) put customer needs first; and (3) move quickly to implement new strategies. Every day spent waiting to confirm trends before taking a new direction is going to be very costly.

STRATEGIES FOR PROVIDERS, HMOs, AND SUPPLIERS

All major players in the healthcare market—providers, HMOs, and suppliers—should heed this advice:

Consolidation

Everywhere, it seems, there are announcements of the formation of networks, joint ventures, and regional and statewide integrated delivery networks. This game of musical chairs may not have enough seats for all participants. Those who consolidate now can make their market and assure their future.

Timing

The time is *now* for America's hospitals, physicians, health systems, and healthcare suppliers to combine to form new and innovative delivery systems. The players must not fall victim to the "paralysis of analysis," deferring choices while others make the first moves. The best partnerships will be the combinations of "strong plus strong" organizations that recognize their mutual need and the advantages of alignment.

Bias for Action

This is the ground floor of twenty-first century healthcare. Providers, HMOs, and suppliers: wait no longer. The window of opportunity is closing, and the time for change is dawning. The American sixth stage of U.S. healthcare market evolution will be here by the millenium.

SOURCES

Anders, G. "Hospitals' Push to Shorten Patient Stays May Have Hit Its Limit, Study Suggests," *Wall Street Journal,* 2 May 1996, p. B6.

Bader, B. 1996. "The 'Grand Experiment': The Meridia Health System/Blue Cross Venture." *Health System Leader* 3 (1): 19–27.

Bergman, R. 1994. "Health Care in a Wired World." *Hospitals & Health Networks* 68 (16): 28–36

Burda, D. 1994a. "Former Charleston, S.C. Rivals Open Dialogue on Affiliation." *Modern Healthcare* 24 (32): 62–64.

———. 1994b. "Geisinger Ruling May Mean Fewer Tax Exemptions." *Modern Healthcare* 24 (32): 40, 58.

Cochrane, J. 1993. "The Ultimate Model for Integrated Healthcare?" *Integrated Healthcare Report* 2 (10): 8–11.

Coile, R., and H. L. Menkin. 1996. *A View of the Future: Competition, Capitation, Consolidation and Cooperation.* Sacramento, CA: California Healthcare Association.

Freudenheim, M. "Health Industry Is Changing Itself Ahead of Reform," *New York Times,* 27 June 1994, pp. A1, C4.

Goldsmith, J. C. 1994. "The Illusive Logic of Integration." *Healthcare Forum Journal* 37 (5): 26–31.

Greenberg, D. S. "Health Reform is Happening Anyway," *Baltimore Sun,* 23 October 1994, p. B1.

Group Health Cooperative. 1993. "HMO Employer Data and Information: A Special Report Measuring Utilization, Quality and Value at Group Health Cooperative." Seattle, WA. September; cited in *Capitation I: The New American Medicine.* 1994. Washington, DC: The Governance Committee, Advisory Board.

Hamer, R. 1996. "HMO Industry Report." *InterStudy Competitive Edge* 6 (1): 1–136.

Henderson, J. A. 1995. "Life After Reform: Health Providers and Suppliers Readjust in 1995." *SMG Market Letter* 9 (1): 1–8.

———. 1996. "Aligned Missions of MCOs and IHNs Spark Alliances." *SMG Market Letter* 10 (5): 1–2.

Lafuente, D. 1994. "California Health Network Recruits Three New Systems." *Modern Healthcare* 24 (21): 8.

Lumsdon, K., and M. Haglund. 1994. "For-Profits: The Right Medicine for Some Markets?" *Hospitals & Health Networks* 68 (12): 34–42.

Lutz, S. 1994. "Groups Form Desktop Health Networks." *Modern Healthcare* 24 (32): 66–70.

———. 1996. "Arizona Mega-System Weighs Partners." *Modern Healthcare* 26 (29): 10.

Lutz, S., and E. P. Gee. 1995. *The For-Profit Healthcare Revolution: The Growing Impact of Investor-Owned Health Systems in America.* Chicago: Irwin Professional Publishing.

McManis, G. 1994. "The New Delivery and Financing Realities." *Hospitals & Health Networks* 68 (16): 38–42.

Melville, B. 1994. "Copying Minneapolis–St. Paul Hospitals Could Save $12B A Year." *Health Care Competition Week* 11 (2): 1–2.

Miller, J. 1995a. "Coastal's North Carolina HMO Starts Up and Florida IPA Joint Venture Is Launched." *Integrated Healthcare Report* 4 (1): 15.

———. 1995b. "Integrated Healthcare Information Systems." *Integrated Healthcare Report* 4 (1): 1–11.

———. 1995c. "May Enters Into Arizona Joint Venture with John Alden." *Integrated Healthcare Report* 3 (1): 15.

Morrison, I., and G. Schmid. 1994. *Future Tense: The Business Realities of the Next Ten Years.* New York: William Morrow and Co.

New York Times. "State Officials Strive to Bring the Health Care Debate Home." 25 September 1994, p. 13.

Olmos, D. R. "Appetite for Expansion: The Changing Healthcare Industry," *Los Angeles Times*, 21 February 1995, pp. D1, D3.

Rovner, J. 1996. "Should Providers Run Their Own HMOs?" *Health System Leader* 3 (1): 4–11.

Sandrick, K. 1994. "Washington, DC: The Capital's A Company Town, But the Company's Not Quite There Yet." *Hospitals & Health Networks* 68 (12): 60–64.

Sardinha, C. 1995. "Price Cuts Help Medica Win Market Share and Improve Risk Selection." *Managed Care Outlook* 8 (2): 1–2.

Scott, L. 1994. "Affiliation Boom, Battle for County Hit K.C." *Modern Healthcare* 24 (32): 138–44.

Sherer, J. 1994. "Strategy by Analogy." *Hospitals & Health Networks* 68 (12): 58–59.

Unland, J. J. 1994. "Hospital-Physician Relationships in the Managed Care Environment." *Journal of Medical Practice Management* 10 (1): 6–10.

Index

Academic medical centers, 73, 189–90, 215, 225
   and hub-and-spoke models, 97, 190
   and satellite networks, 112, 189
Access Health (CA), 76
Access managers, 76–77
   See also Gatekeepers
Access points, consumer, 76, 83, 106, 116, 123
Accountability, performance, 138
Administrative costs, economies of scale in, 33–34
Administrative costs, reducing, 15, 177–78, 180
   by centralization, 142
   by HMO competitors, 85, 90, 139
   by merged HMOs, 30–31, 32
   cooperative integration for, 37
   to preserve profits, 2

Adventist Health System/West (CA), 12, 138, 140, 212
Advisory Board Company, 44, 64, 67, 69
Advocate Health (IL), 91, 140, 158, 162
Aetna, 31, 32, 33, 35, 157
   acquisition of providers, 7, 143, 157, 182
   and health promotion, 219
   as managed care plan, 10
   as network manager, 158
   and physician networks, 29
   and staff-model employment, 113, 182
Aetna/U.S. Healthcare, 32, 182, 215
Affiliated Medical Center (MN), 223
Alegent Health (NE), 182
Allegiance LLC (MI), 93
Alliant Health System (KY), 140
Allina (MN), 35, 91, 130, 203
   governing board, 201

Index

and integration, 14, 36, 222, 223
Allina Health System/Medica (MN), 86
Alta Bates Health System (CA), 140
Alta Bates Medical Center, 184
Alternative therapies, 17, 145
Ambulatory services, 4, 7, 105, 167, *180*
 for chronic care, 70
 and inpatient reduction, 1, *12*, 13, 122–23
 in primary care, 103, 112, 162
 in regional centers, 15
American Association of PHOs/Integrated Healthcare Delivery Systems, 88
American Group Practice Association, 52
American Healthcare Systems, 99, 203
American Hospital Association, 4, 84, 147, 151, 159
American Medical Association, 3, 84, 96, 126
American Medical International, 141, 213
Anchor (IL), 35
Anderson, David, 82
Anthem, 31
Antitrust issues, 75, 129, 131–32, 147
Arnwine, Don L., 169
Aspen Medical Group (MN), 14, 130, 203, 221
Aspen Plus Health Network (MN), 203
Associated Group of Indianapolis, 31, 187
Attorneys, roles of, 2, 11

Aurora Health Network (WI), 186

Baltimore Medical Group (MD), 127–28
Baptist Health System (AR), 140, 191
Bargaining power, 114
Barkley, Ronald, 171
Barnes-Jewish-Christian Health System (MO), 10, 97, 99, 199
Barton, Ray, 112, 184
Baxter Healthcare, 96, 116
Baylor Health Care System (TX), 91, 220
Bay Physicians Medical Group (CA), 184
Bay Shores Medical Group (CA), 126
Bay State (MA), 126
Behavioral Health Direct (IL), 158
Behavioral health services, 158
Benchmarking, 7, 94, 146
Blue Cross (AR), 191
Blue Cross (MI), 145
Blue Cross (MN), 130, 203
Blue Cross (NJ), 182, 215, 220
Blue Cross:
 capital reserves of, 15
 mergers, 30–31
 partnerships, 14
 and physician networks, 29
Blue Cross/Blue Shield (MN):
 acquisition of providers, 221
 and employer contracts, 86
 and out-of-state markets, 223
 provider network, 221
Blue Cross/Blue Shield (NJ), 29, 31, 113
Blue Cross/Blue Shield (OH), 142, 185

Index

Blue Cross/Blue Shield (OR), 217
Blue Cross/Blue Shield, 5, 33, 187–89
 consolidations, 30–31
 merger agreements, 187
 and physician-hospital organizations (PHOs), 87
 and point-of-service plans, 30
 in provider-payer partnerships, 142–43
Blues plans:
 competitive strategies, 143
 Indiana, 31, 187
 Kentucky, 187
 and managed care, 33, 188
 National Accounts Consortium, 31
 New England, 187, 189
 Ohio, 31, 187
Boards, health system, 51, 202–03
Boland, Peter, 13
Boland Healthcare, 12–13
Bond, Charles, 114–15
Bon Secours-St. Francis Xavier (SC), 220
Boone Hospital Center (MO), 97
Branick, Robert, 93
Brighton Medical Center (ME), 10
Brim (OR), 142
Bundled fees, 4, 47
Burry, John, 185
Business Health Care Action Group (BHCAG), 86
Buyers Health Care Action Group (MN), 148

California Department of Health Services, 107
California Healthcare Association, 224
California Healthcare System, 12, 140, 212
California Health Network (CHN), 12, 137, 140, 212
California Health Systems, 152
California Medical Association, California Advantage, 34
California Pacific Medical Center, 93
California Pacific Medical Services, 93
California Patient Protection Act, 22
California Public Employees Retirement System (CalPERS), 28, 138, 185, 190
Cancer Network, National Comprehensive, 161
Capacity, excess, 151–52, 180, 192, 223–24
Capital, 73, 145, 150, 172
Capital investments, 4, 203–05, 222
 by hospitals, 66, 101–02, 162
 in integrated delivery networks (IDNs), 196
 for statewide networks, 146
Capitalization, 152
 by management service organizations, 114
 for clinics without walls, 129
 for independent physician organizations, 122
 for physician-hospital organizations, 51, 95, 139
 for regional networks, 11
Capital reserves, 14–15, 32, 73
Capitated plans, 44

Index

Capitation, 41–80, *50*, 101, *102*
　advantages of, 48, 49, 59
　contracts, *51*, *68*, 83
　for controlling HMO costs, 2, 28–29, 49
　and decreased utilization, 15, 28, 42–43
　defined, 41–42, 46
　as dominant form of payment, 16, 41–42, 44
　full-risk, *68*, 72–75, 88
　global contracts, 96, 102, 138, 143, 157, 179
　and group practices, *52*
　incentives, progressive, 77–78, 98
　and managed care triad, 179, *180*
　for Medicaid benefits, 25, 54–55
　subspecialty, 75
　and trust, mutual, 50
Capitation management, 224
Capitation rates, 53
　per member per month, 46, 108
　for specialists, *76*
CareAmerica, 3
CareData Reports, 95
CareLink (WV), 51
CareMark International, 96, 116, 122, 144, 172, 224
Caremark/MedPartners, 96, 200
Carle Clinic (IL), 162
Carlson, Ed, 15
Carveouts, 47, 144, 189–90
　mental health services as, 57
　niche, 69–70
Case management, 25, 58, *180*
　centralized, 67
　continuous, 16, 71, 76–77
　primary care, 89, 106

Catholic Health Association, 217
Catholic Healthcare West (CA), 12, 115, 183
Centers of excellence, 69, 161
Certificate-of-need, 220
Charleston Area Medical Center (WV), 51
Charleston Hospital (WV), 51
Chasin, Beth, 92
Childbirth, 22, 63, 97, 163
Children's Hospital (CA), 93
Chronic care, 70, 76, 106
　capitation of, *68*, 70–71
　management of, 90–91, 106, 157
Cigna (PA), 5, 31, *33*, 34, 90, 218
　carveout contracting, 189–90
　primary care networks, 143
　staff-model clinics, 96, 111
Cleveland Clinic, 185, 197, 198
Cleveland Health Network (OH), 220
Cleveland Health Quality Choice project, 10, 186
Clinical paths, 11, *12*, 15, 90, 108, 175, 216
Clinics without walls, components of, 128–30
Clinton, Bill, President, 84, 147
Clinton, Hillary Rodham, and health reform, 2–3, 23
Coastal Healthcare Group (NC), 220
Coastal Physician Group, 143
Cochrane, John D., 186
Codman, E.A., 162–63
Collaboration, hospital-physician, 169–70

Index

Colorado Division of Insurance, 187
Columbia/HCA Healthcare, 140, 141–43
 and brand name marketing, 212–13
 and consolidation, 6–7
 in joint ventures, 172, 215, 220
 mergers/acquisitions, 146, 185, 215, 219
 on stock exchange, 200
 and payer contracts, 156
Columbia/HCA/HealthTrust, 143
Columbia-Presbyterian Medical Center (NY), 200
Columbia Regional Hospital (MO), 97
Commanche Regional Medical Center (OK), 57
Commerce, U.S. Department of, and national health expenditures, 122
Commercial lives, 22
Communication, 152
Community health clinics, 219
Community health information networks, 58, 142, 150–51, 216
Community Health Systems of Houston, 141
Community Hospitals of Indianapolis, 8
Community Memorial Hospital, 159
Community Mutual (OH), 33, 187
Community Mutual Insurance of Cincinnati, 31
Community service, 145, 191, 203

McGaw, Foster G., Prize for, 112
Competition, 35
Competition, managed, 98, 161
 for control of markets, 11–13
 and direct contracting, 158
 and price pressures, 1
Competition:
 market, 179
 nonprofits, 12
 on performance, 214, 215
Competition, price, 27–28, 32
 and annual rate increase, 225
 for integrated systems, 142
 in metropolitan areas, 22, 77
 "predatory pricing," 27
 and profitability, 190
 traditional insurance plans, 24
Competition, provider networks vs. managed care, 36–37
Computer linkages, physician-hospital, 170–71
 See also Information systems
Consolidation, 1, 2, 81, 195, 226
 accelerated rate of, 6, 32, 35
 of managed care plans, 14–15
 provider, 147
 regional, 13, 98
 of support functions, 205
Consortium Research on Indicators of System Performance, 91
Consumer price index, 23, 27, 178
Contracting, direct, 9, 114, 157–59

Index

and integrated delivery
networks, 92, 195
and integrated delivery
systems, 138
with payers, 83, 158
physician-hospital
organizations, 86–
88, 87, 88–89, 139
physician management
corporations, 96
single service, 158
Cook, Quentin, 137
Copayments, consumer, 25,
53, 62
Cornell Medical Center (NY),
200
Cornell University/New York
Hospital, 97
Corporate-practice laws,
148–49
Costs of services, 13, 116, 210
clinical care, 16, 83, 181
data availability on, 16, 216
management of, 89, 124
Credentialing, 164
by clinics without walls, 130
by management service
organizations, 114
of health system boards,
202–03
provider, 15, 37, 59, 89, 92,
110
Crimmins, Tim, 83
Curtin, Leah, 115
Customer satisfaction, 94, 123,
184, 186, 205, 216
Customer service, 31, 48, 180
integration and, 37, 92
measurement of, 94

Dakota Clinic (ND), 223
Dartmouth Medical School
(NH), 91
Daughters of Charity Health
System/West (CA), 12
Davidson, Jack, 191
Decentralization, 111
Decision making:
in for-profit settings, 200
participation in, 168
See also Governance
Delivery, service, 15, 31, 34
Delivery systems, 73–75, 113
staff-model, 32, 113, 131,
191
See also Integrated delivery
systems
Deloitte & Touche physician
survey, 36
Dental care, 69
Diagnostics, 42, 46, 47, 65,
180
Disease management, 90–91,
175
cost effective, 157
Doctors Health Plan (FL),
96–97, 97
Doctors Health Plan (NC),
220
Downey Community Hospital
(CA), 66–67
Drisner, Robert, 159
Drugs:
benefits for, consumer, 25,
62
costs of, prescription, 63,
211
Due diligence, 214

Economies of scale, 33–34
Economy, healthcare, national
expenditures for, 123
Efficiency, clinical, 173–74
by facilities/services closure,
146
and capitation, 42, 46
emphasis on, 13, 29, 91

and integration, 98
and profitability, 43
EHS Health Care (IL), 140
Ellwood, Paul, 203
Emerald, 10
Emergency services, 55, 63, 75, *180*, 181
EmoryCare, 190
Emory Clinic, 189
Emory University (GA), 6, 190
Empire (NY), *33*, 187
Employee Retirement Income Security Act of 1974, 137
Employer coalitions, *12*, 185–86
  of health plans, 137
  and integration, 15
  in regional markets, 147–48
Employers, *87*, 137
  benefit negotiations, 84
  cost consciousness of, 177
  as network managers, 185–86
  preference for managed care, 24
  self-insured, 85
Enrollment, 23, 24, 27
  in capitated plans, 44, 62, 77
  declining, 85
  in Medicaid, 25
  in physician-hospital organizations, 89
  projections, *21*
  in regional plans, 140–41
Epic Healthcare, 141, 213
Equity, 145, 184
Equity opportunities, 16, 177, 183–84, 191
  Columbia/HCA, 142, 200
  HealthEast, 222
  PacifiCare, 156
  in physician-owned networks, 179

Estes Park Institute, 164
Ethix Northwest Seattle, 31
Everett Clinic (WA), 53
ExclusiCare (NE), 182

Fairview-HealthEast-University (MN), 14
Fairview Health System (MN), 86, 97–98, 128, 203, 222
Fallon Clinic (MA), 125–26, 183, 197, 198
Fallon Community Health Plan (MA), 63
Fargo Clinic (ND), 162
Federal Trade Commission, 75, 132, 147
Fee-for-service, 53, 64
  and fragmented care, 42
  modified system, 86
  networks, 32, 36
  payments, 41, 47, 55, 133
  for specialists, *45*, 49, *76*
Fees, discounted, 27, 37, 62, 85, 110, 124
FHP International (CA), 29, *33*
  and consolidation, 15
  and employer pressure, 185
  increase in premiums, 28
  mergers, 200
  on stock exchange, 27
  strategic alliance, 217–18
Fine, Allen, 51
First Option (NJ), 214–15
Florida Hospital, 213
Florida Independent Physicians Association, 220
Ford, Dan, 133
Foundation Health (CA), 29, 157, 183
  and consolidation, 15
  premiums for, 3, *5*
Foundations, medical, 16, *51*, 64, 138

Index

creation of, 149, 171, 183
tax-exempt, 155, 218
Friendly Hills Healthcare Network (CA), 143, 144
Friendly Hills Medical Group (CA), 50, 105, 116
Future Tense (Morrison; Schmidt), 224

Gatekeepers, 25, 47, 75–76
  cardiology, 64–65, 156
  nurses as, 115
Gatekeepers, primary care, 29, 107, 130, 162
  capitated, 102
  for clinics without walls, 130
  in integrated health systems, 116
Geisinger Clinic (PA), 126, 145, 197, 198
Geisinger Foundation, 218
General Health System (LA), 215
Geographic coverage, 73, 127, 145, 157, 222
Geriatric Health Systems (CA), 58
Gingrich, Newt, 3, 26
Glatstein, Harry R., 158
Global fees, 47
Goldsmith, Jeff C., 149–50, 166, 217
Goldstein, Doug, 92
Governance, 149, 195–207
  by cooperation, 164–66, 205–06
  of clinics, 197–98
  cooperation in, 205
  in hub-and-spoke model, 159, 160, 198
  models for, 197–202
  physicians role in, 173, 196–97
  shared, 16, 169, 184, 204, 222
  structures, 124, 127
Government intervention, 182, 185, 187
Government regulation, 169, 205
  corporate-practice laws, 148–49
  of insurance companies, 85
  of managed care, 22, 31
  merger guidelines, 131
  of provider prices, 221
  See also Antitrust issues
Grab, Edward, 54
Graduate Health System (PA), 91, 200
Greater Baltimore Medical Center, 9
Greater Southeast, 212
Green, Roger, 86–87
Group Health Association (RI), 187
Group Health Association of America:
  enrollment statistics, 24, 178
  on economies of scale, 33–34
  on physician-hospital organizations, 88
  on point-of-service plans, 30
  on provider-sponsored networks, 85
Group Health Cooperative of Puget Sound (WA), 63, 211
  administrative costs, 213–14
  as nonprofit plan, 23
  in strategic alliance, 124, 201
Group practice without walls, 109, 126–28, 162
Group purchasing, 67, 114, 160

Index

Guardian (NY), 33
Gulf South Health Plans, 215

Hallmark Healthcare, 141
Halvorsen, George, 14
Hamilton/KSA (GA), 52
Harris Methodist Health Plan (TX), 140–41
Hartshorn, Terry, 103
Harvard Community Health Plan (MS), 5, 124, 187
Hatch, Stephen W., 108
Hays, Patrick, 111
Health Advantage (AR), 191
Health and Hospitals Corporation (NY), 200
Health and Human Services, U.S. Department of, 25
Health Capital Group, 218
Health Care Advisory Group, 93
Healthcare Association of Southern California, 151
Health Care Financing Administration, 24, 27
 and Medicaid contracting, 54–55, 71, 79, 82
 Medicare guidelines, 25
Health Care Group, 54
Health Care Partners (CA), 126
Health Care Service (IL), 33
Health Central (MN), 203
HealthEast system (MN), 86–87, 203, 222
Health First Medical Group (TN), 113
Health Insurance Association of America, 85
Health maintenance organizations, 87
 acquisition of providers, 35–36, 113, 117–18, 124–25, 192
 bankruptcies in, 86–87
 certification for, 79
 comparative data on, 186, 216
 consumer-owned, 221
 disadvantages of, 85
 disenrollment rates, 77
 enrollment in, 127, 178
 as intermediaries, 84, 85, 139
 licensing for, 85, 86, 126, 145
 as long-term investment, 27
 medical loss ratios, 38, 85
 Medicare-qualified, 22
 as network managers, 82, 181–82
 patient preference in, 26
 profits for, 27–28, 32–34
 provider-sponsored, 34, 36, 61, 96, 126, 214
 regulation of, 86
 reserve requirements for, 86, 87
 staff-model, 144–45
 treatment guidelines for, 89
 See also Managed care
Health Midwest (MO), 219
HealthOne (MN), 221
Health-OnLine, 216–17
HealthPartners (AZ), 92, 219
HealthPartners (MN), 14, 203
 acquisition of providers, 221
 and direct contracting, 86
 and market domination, 130
 in partnerships, 148
HealthPartners Health Plan (AZ), 36
Health Partners of Southern Arizona, 92
Health Plan of Greater San Diego, 126
Health plans, 33, 137

Index

Health promotion, 57–58, *180*
  benefits of, 218–19
  premium rebates in, 211
  primary care in, 103
HealthSource (NH), 190, 191
HealthSpan (MN), 14, 36, 128, 203, 221–22
HealthSystem Minnesota, 148
Health Systems International, 14–15
HealthTrust, 141, 213
Healthy Options (WA), 55
Heartland Health Systems (KS), 35
HEDIS indicators, 18, 59, 77, 164, 215
Henderson, John A., 11, 13
Hennepin County Medical Society (MN), 128
Henry Ford Health System (MI), 167
  primary care networks, 116, 130–31
  and report card, 91
  and statewide expansion, 145
  and telemedicine linkage, 215
Highline Community Hospital (WA), 55
Hill-Burton Act, 223
Hillman, Jim, 126
Hill Medical Group (CA), 115
HIP (NY), 23, 26
HMO Arkansas, 191
HMO Blue, 143
Holy Cross Hospital (MD), 9
Home health services, 69
Horizon Healthcare (WI), 159
Hospice services, 70–71
Hospital chains, for-profit, 141–42
Hospital Corporation of America, 213
Hospitalizations, 42, *46*, 47, 62, 98
Hospital networks, nonprofit, 139–41
Hospitals:
  assets of, 66
  brand name chains of, 212–13
  capital investments by, 66, 162
  capitation for, 49, *102*
  closure of, 146, 196, 222
  and flexible staffing, 66
  and group practice development, 162
  independence of, 6
  management personnel in, 66
  marketing to purchasers, 66
  and national health expenditures, *123*
  as network managers, 182–83
  networks of, 9–10, 11, 16
  per diem payments for, 29, 36, 41, 69, 88
  discounted rate for, 67, 179
  and physician acquisition, 162
  primary care division in, 110–11
  specialty care in, 69–70, 75, 77
  surplus beds in, 151, 223–24, 225
  See also Providers
Hospitals and Health Networks, 13–14, 52
Hough, Douglas, 141
Houston Healthcare Purchasing Organization, 8
Hub-and-spoke models, 180

Index

and academic medical centers, 97, 142, 179, 190
as cancer networks, 161
governance of, 159, 160, 198, 198–99
as regional delivery systems, 159–60
Humana (KY), 33, 35, 78, 217
Huntington Provider Group, 50

Incentive funds. *See* Risk pools
Incentives:
for integration, 42
for networks, 196
performance, 142, 181
shared, 167
Indemnity plans, 24, 48, 143, 188, 190
Independent Health Association (NY), 191
Independent physician organizations, 121–34
characteristics of, 122
practice guidelines for, 124, *180*
Independent practice associations:
costs of, 171
management of, 115
and multispecialty clinics, 162
and physician-hospital organizations, 51
physician-sponsored, 11, 144
support services for, 112
Independent practice associations, 108
Inflation, medical cost, 1, 27, 177–78
Information network, *180*
Information systems, 92
community health, 58, 142, 150–51, 197, 215
compatibility in, 138, 146, 173
computerized, 8, 16, 66, 83, 86, 91
contract management software, 8
data collection, 73, 86
demographic, 104
integrated, 37
key issues for, 150
limitations in, 124, 158
management, 129
outcome predictive, 91
and profitability, 122
shared, 32, 85
Inpatient services, declining use of, 62–64, *63*, 224
with capitation, *43*, 44–45, 67
changed treatment emphasis and, 13
episodes of care program and, 90
with managed care, *46*, *63*
Inpatient services, specialty care, *180*
Institute for Clinical Systems Integration, 148
Insurance, 85, 86
Insurance, commercial plans, 5, *87*, 185
acquisition of providers, 113, 179
Insurers as network managers, 181–82
Integra Health System (AZ), 219
Integrated delivery networks, 11–13, 81–99, 195
components of, 83
conflict of interest in, 204–05

239

Index

decentralized, 105, 111, 146
governance models for, 197–202
and management service organizations, 92, 114
in post-reform environment, 195–207
roles of, 93–94
Integrated delivery systems, 16, *51*, 113, 127–28
advantages of, 138, 159
development of, 143–44
nonprofit, 6
purchasing power of, 13
staff-model HMOs as, 144
structure of, 13
and system capitation, 74, 78
and "virtual integration," 150, 217–18
"Integrated service clusters," 112
Integrated service networks, 13–14
accreditation for, 139
development of, 148
for Medicaid contracts, 221
Integration, 36–37, 110
InterMountain HealthCare, 141, 215
Internal Revenue Service, 94, 204
and 501(c)(3) status, 23, 95, 96, 144, 218
InterStudy, 34, 203
and capitation, 44, 55
and for-profit HMOs, 62
growth statistics from, 22, 56
and point-of-service plans, 29–30
and provider-sponsored HMOs, 214

Jamplis, Robert, 42
Japsen, Bruce, 96
Jayhawk Alliance, 219
John Alden Life Insurance, 218
John Deere Health Plan, 5
Johns Hopkins University Hospital (MD), 9, 73
Johns Hopkins HealthCare System (MD), 78, 88, 127, 199
Johns Hopkins Hospital, 9
Joint Commission on Accreditation of Healthcare Organizations, 4, 139
Joint practice organization, 112
Joint ventures, 30, 36, 78, 92–93, 147, 198
academic medical centers in, 97
for-profit with nonprofit entities, 172
in physician-hospital integration, 155
provider-payer, 185
for statewide provider networks, 141
Justice, U.S. Department of, 75, 147

Kaiser Health Plan, 142–43, 173, 185, 218–19
Kaiser Permanente (CA), 5, 33, 167, 173
as a staff-model HMO, 26, 44, 144–45, 213–14, 217
expansion of, 7
integration of, 74
in joint ventures, 198
nonprofit competition for, 12
nonprofit status, 23
premium reductions, 138

in primary care, 104
and restructuring, 15
in statewide partnerships, 142–43
Kaiser Permanente Medical Group, 104
Kansas Medical Society, 35
Kaufman, Nathan, 88, 157
Kimmel, Alan, 127
KPMG–Peat Marwick, 23, 82

Laboratory services, 46, 77, 142
Lahey Clinic (MS), 124, 147, 197
Lang, Daniel A., 164
Langness, David, 62
Large Employer Initiative (MN), 221
Larkovich, Andrew, 126
Leadership, 94, 167–69, 202–03
Legacy Health System (OR), 217
Liability, limiting, 48, 54, 84
Liberty HealthCare System (NJ), 92
LifeSpan (MN), 221
Loma Linda University Medical Center (CA), 12, 140, 212
Long-term care, subacute, 70
Lord, Jonathan T., 4
Los Angeles Times, 3
Lovelace Clinic (NM), 90, 111, 218
Loyola University Medical Center (IL), 78
Lutheran General Health Plan, 162
Lutheran General HealthSystem (IL), 140

Maine Medical Center, 10

Managed care, 169, 177
academic medical centers in, 97
competing forms of, 88
contracting, 129, 179
conversion to, 33, 143, 182, 185
discounted fees for, 47–48
employers preference for, 24
government regulation of, 22, 31
infrastructure, 138, 157
networks, costs of, 171
opposition to, 17–18
physicians signed to, 23
in post-reform marketplace, 178, 195–207
staff, experienced in, 73, 145
stages of, 3–16, 5
Management, 8, 73, 94
capitation, 224
centralized, 149
of chronic care, 70–71, 90–91, 106, 157
clinical, 16, 173
efficiencies in, 213–14
of financial risk, 150
medical directors in, 73, 89, 169
network, costs of, 15
practice, 129
resource, 74
shared, 205
See also Network management
Management service organizations, 16, *51*, 92, 101
costs of, 171
and integrated delivery networks, 92

Index

as network managers, 183–84
physician's organizations as, 73–74
provider-owned, 113–15, 114
roles of, 72, 93–94
Managers:
chief information officer, 216
experienced, 133, 145, 222
vice president for medical care, 173
Maricopa County Hospital (AZ), 215
Market:
advantage, 13, 143
forces, 1, 36, 37
leverage, 81, 82, 88, 91–92, 97
opportunities, 75, 83, 212
post-reform, 13
target, 137
trends, 2–3, 24–35
Marketing:
brand name, 12, 32, 212–13, 218
by health plans, 12, *180*
by hospitals, 66
by providers, 92
costs of, 48
group, 129
Markets, 5
advanced, 3–4, 17, 62
domination of, 32, 101
emerging, 127
geographic, 132
Marketshare, 32, 85
Marshfield Clinic (WI), 126
Mary Hitchcock Health System (NH), 91
Mason, Stephen, 140
Massachusetts General/Brigham, 189

Massachusetts General Hospital, 124
Massachusetts Rate Setting Commission, 27
Mayerhofer, John, 48
Mayo Clinic (MN), 145, 189, 197–98, 218, 219
Mayo Healthcare Network, 218
McCann, Richard, 223
McGaw, Foster G., 112
McKell, Doug C., 116, 121, 123
McKemy, Victoria, 156
McManis, Gerald, 83
M.D. Anderson (TX), 161
MedCenters Health Plan, 14
Medica (MN), 14, 36, 203, 222
Medicaid, 2, 22, 34, 177, 221
block grant funding for, 3
capitated, 34, 54–55, 212
contracting, 15, 82, 106, 199–200
and managed care, 23, 24–25, 82, 140
primary care services for, 25
programs, large, 137
reform initiatives, 148–49, 212
MediCal (CA), 107–08
Medical Care America (FL), 213
Medical Network of New Mexico (Med-Net), 112
Medical University of South Carolina, 142
Medicare, 22, 25–26, 34
below-inflation payments, 2
capitation contracting, 34, 55–57, 71–72, 79
and managed care, 23, 25, 61–62, 82, 140, 187
risk contracting, *68*, 71–72

Index

Medlantic HealthCare Group, 212
MedPartners (AL), 96, 144
MedPartners/Mullikin (AL), 122, 126, 224
Memorial Sloan-Kettering Memorial Center (NY), 161
Menorah (MO), 219
Mental health services, 47
  capitation model in, 57, 69
Mercy Healthcare of Phoenix, 219
Mercy Health System (MI), 91
Mercy Health System (NY), 191
Mercy Hospital (ME), 10
Mercy Medical Center (IA), 215
Mergers:
  asset-based, 150, 196
  economy-driven, 140
  as "mega-mergers," 186–87
  noncash, 183
  payer-provider, 74, 128, 214
  physician, 131–32
  and statewide networks, 146–47
  See also Consolidation
Mergers/acquisitions, 23
  accelerations in, 32
  candidates for, 14
Meridia Health System (OH), 10, 142, 184–85
Meridia Health System/Blue Cross (OH), 220
Merry, Martin D., 167–68
Methodist Hospital (IN), 109
Methodist Hospital (MN), 130, 148, 221
Methodist Hospitals of Dallas, 220
Metrahealth, 32
Metropolitan Life (NY), 32, *33*
Meyer Medical Group, 189

Micromanagement:
  of healthcare usage, 2, 29
  of provider performance, 79, 206
Mid-America Health First, 219
Middle Tennessee Network, 183
Miles, John, 131, 132
Miller, Wayne J., 148
MinnesotaCare, 221
Minnesota Employers Association, 223
Minnesota Medical Association, 128
Modern Healthcare, 51, 88, 96
Monitors, in-home, 16
Montgomery General Hospital (MD), 9
Mount Sinai Health System, 92
Mount Sinai Medical Center (OH), 10
M Plan (IN), 109
Mullikin Medical Group (CA), 103–04, 223–24
MultiCare Health System (WA), 34
Multispecialty groups, 12, 159, 162, 189
  acquisition of, 9
  primary care emphasis, 111, 181
Muris, Tom, 26
Mutual of Omaha (NE), *33*, 182

Nathanson, Philip, 219
National Association of Physician-Hospital Organizations, 108
National Household Interview Survey, 104
National Medical Enterprises, 141, 147, 213

243

Index

Network:
 capitalization of, 11
 capitation, 73–74
 credentialing, streamlined, 31
 ownership, 181–82, 196
Networking:
 by hospitals, 9–10
 and partnership selection, 145–46
Network management, 15
 as bureaucracy, 149–50
 by HMOs, 82
 by insurers, 82
 by providers, 92
 and coordinator, *180*
 costs of, 15, 59
Networks:
 Blues provider, 187, 189
 clinical, 66, 128–30, 161
 fee-for-service, 32
 local, 138
 multicenter, 199
 primary care, 90, 101–17
 primary care satellite, 112
 provider-sponsored, 83–85
 of public hospitals, 199–200
Networks, regional, *12*, 138, 179, 183
 brand name chains in, 212–13
Networks, statewide, 16, 50, 91, 137–53
 development of, 141–42, 146–47, 211–12
 models for, 139–45
 stakeholders in, 152
New England Journal of Medicine, 23
New York Hospital, 97
New York Life Insurance, 29
Norling, Rick, 222
Northeast Ohio Community Health Plan, 223

North Memorial Hospital (MN), 222
Northwest Community Hospital (IL), 140
Northwestern Community Hospital (IL), 35
Northwestern Health Care Network (IL), 35, 91, 140
Northwest Medical Center (MD), 9
Nursing:
 facilities, *123*
 in primary care delivery, 115–16
 skilled, *102*, 156
Nursing Management, 115

Occupational health services, 69, 116
Ochsner Clinic (LA), 145, 197, 198
O'Hare, Patrick, 95
Omni Health Plan (CA), 183
Oregon Medical Group, 162
Orlando Regional Medical Center (FL), 213
Orlikoff, James E., 94, 162, 202
OrNda (TN), 141, 146, 213, 220
Out-of-area coverage, 84, 140
Outsourcing, 144
Overhead, reducing, 32–33, 59, 114, 144, 181

PacifiCare (CA), 56, 103, 156, 185
 and consolidation, 15
 expansion of, 7, 62
 increase in premiums, 28
 Medicare contracting, 56
 and multi-year contracts, 217
 on stock exchange, 27

Index

Pacific Business Group on Health, 28, 148, 186
Pacific Employers Group, 185
Pacific Medical Services, 93
Pacific Physician Services (CA), 147
Palo Alto Clinic Foundation, 42
Panels, provider, 55, 73, 82, 89
Park Nicollet Clinic (MN), 130, 148, 221
Partners Community Healthcare (MA), 126
Partners Health Plan (AZ), 36
Partnerships, 145–46, 178, 192, 226
   academic medical centers with insurers, 189–90
   communication in, 152–53
   community, 201–02
   as network managers, 184–85
   provider, 155–75, 214–15
Partnerships, provider with payer, 142–43, 177–92, 191, 200–201
   key factors in, 214
Partnerships:
   public-private, 215
   triad-model, 184
   virtual integration and, 217–18
Patient-centered care, 145
Patient outcomes, assessment of, 83, 123, 163, 181
   from available data, 216
   for chronic care, 71
   for continuous improvement, 94
Patients:
   disabled, 57
   disadvantaged, 106, 107, 112–13, 219
   management of, 83, 106
   population of, 83, 84, 91, 223
   profiles of, 53
   uninsured, 14, 106, 212, 221
Patient satisfaction, 216
Payers:
   competitive strengths of, 12, 32
   demands on providers, 12
   as future network managers, 190–92
   insurance, indemnity, 23, 24, 27, 38
   insurance, traditional, 38
Performance evaluations, 73
   by payer, 8, 10, 13, 18, 24, 32
   by provider, 11, 91
   by purchaser, 8, 10, 18, 86, 163
   and peer review, 164, 167
Performance standards, 85
Perrin, Towers, 34
Pezzoli, Robert, 9
PHP Healthcare, 143
PhyCor (TN), 96, 122, 172, 200
Physician-driven networks, 143–44
Physician-hospital integration, 155–75
Physician-hospital organizations, 108–09, 172–73
   and capitation, 50, 78, 88
   costs of, 171
   defined, 31, 37
   development of, 51–52, 58, 87
   exclusivity in, 128
   goals of, 138–39
   opposition to, 132–33, 139, 157
   physician leadership in, 64

Index

roles of, 72–73, 73–74, 93–94
as "super-PHOs," 183
as transitional vehicles, 88
under Medicaid capitation, 55
See also Provider-sponsored networks
Physician management corporations, 6, 96–97
as care integrators, 50
Physician networks, criteria for, 107
Physician organizations, 16, 62
open panel independent, 4, 6, 11
Physician Payment Review Commission, 24
Physicians:
autonomy of, 114, 121, 129, 168
consumer's preference, 43
economic control for, 121
and entrepreneurship, 166
equity partnerships for, 142
and fee-for-service, 41, 43, 75, 109, 133, 167
and governance, 173
in managed care agreements, 23, 88, 124–25
and national health expenditures, *123*
as network managers, 183–84, 218
office visits to, 42, *46*
recruitment of, 52–53, 96, 113
See also Primary care physicians; Specialists
Physician Strategies 2000, 101, 116, 121, 123
Piccolo, Lance, 122
Point-of-service plans, *12*, 22, 23, 29–*30*, 38, *188*

Policymakers, congressional, 3, 26
Practice Resource Center, 112
Preferred One (MN), 31–32
Preferred provider designation, seeking, 6
Preferred provider organizations, 4, 31–32, *87*
acquisition of, 145
conversion of, 11, 24
enrollment in, 127
in hub-and-spoke managed care, 159
and marketshare, 186
provider-sponsored, 34–35
PREMERA, 31
Premier Medical Group (CO), 162
Premiums, 3, 190
capitated, 84, 180
disciplined management of, 74
distribution from, 48–49, *50*, 84
rebated, 211
reduced, 2, 27, 138, 178, 185
Presbyterian Healthcare System (TX), 220
Presbyterian Health Plan (NM), 214, 217
as hub-and-spoke model, 218
Preventive care, 91, 103, *180*, 215
Primary care, *180*
as access point, 76, 83, 116, 123
as ambulatory care service, 105, 112, 162
capitation for, 10–11, 48, 56, 75, *102*

Index

capitation rates, 10–11, 43, 108
case managers, 89
defined, 43
revenue per visit, 105
satellite networks, 112
shortage of, 102
Primary care network models, 108–15
Primary care networks, 90, 101–17, 161–62, 179
Primary care networks, development of, 110–11, 116–17
by insurers/HMOs, 9, 29
hospital sponsored, 101–02
Primary care networks, insurer-owned, 113, 183–84
Primary care physicians, 143–44, 181
acquisition of, 8, 116–17, 156, 162
monitoring, 55, 90, 108
role of, 103, 116
Principal Financial Group (IA), 33
Privatization, 23
Profitability, and administrative costs, 139
Profit-sharing, 184
Prospective Payment Assessment Commission, 26
Protocols, 205
clinical treatment, 71, 148, 180
medical, standardized, 11, 15, 59
See also Clinical paths
Provider agreements, exclusive, 137, 177
Providers, 192, 206
and capitation, 28–29, 79
commodification of, 18, 78, 192
competitive strengths of, 12
consultants for, 17, 58, 73
and contracting, at-risk, 174
and cooperation, 18
as plan sponsors, 34–36
reimbursement for, 102, 126
surplus of, 2, 15, 18, 75, 102, 179, 192
See also Hospitals; Physicians
Prudential (NJ), 32, 33, 190
acquisition of providers, 7, 29, 182
employers targeted by, 31
and group practices, 191
in joint ventures, 35
and primary care networks, 143, 157
Prudential Healthcare System, 113
Purchasers, 177
demand for payer premium reductions, 2, 12, 27, 94–95, 185
government, 22, 85
See also Medicaid; Medicare
Purchasing organizations, group, 8, 18, 80, 207
as network managers, 182–83
Purchasing power, 138, 148

Quality:
assessment, 10, 77, 114, 163
continuous improvement in, 110
emphasis on, 8, 124, 186, 205
monitored by provider, 43, 49, 59
Quality assurance, 37, 49, 73, 128, 129
costs of, 15
in-house, 140
and integration, 37, 94

247

Index

Quality data:
  availability of, 216
  on clinical outcomes, 24, 163, 174
  on customer satisfaction, 24
  public report of, 16, 186
Quality management, 66, 146, 162–64, *180*
Qual Med, 5
Quorum Health Resources (TN), 51

Radiology services, *46*, 77
Ramsey County Medical Society (MN), 128
Reform, health, 2–3, 84, 158
  evolutionary, 209–10
  government-sponsored, 24, 71
  market-driven, 21, 61, 221
  models, emerging, for, 210–20
  national, 54–55, 106, 148, 212
  state-level, 13–14, 24, 31–32, 137, 138, 187
Reforming States Group, 212, 212
Reinhardt, Uwe, 27
Reinsurance, 73, 84, 140, *180*
Relationships:
  hospital with physician, 164–66, *165*, 172–74
  medical staff with administration, 166–68
  physician leadership with rank-and-file, 168–69
Religious boundaries, and networks, 8, 9–10, 92, 145, 199
Relman, Arnold, 23
Resurrection Health Care (IL), 78
Revenues, shared, 181
Riece, Richard L., M.D., 108

Rightsizing, 151–52
Risk, acceptance of, 50, 62, 84, 125, 139, 195
Risk, financial, 51, 75, 126, 131, 159
Risk management, 43, 150
  by health promotion, 57–58
  by physician organizations, 16
  by providers, 42, 43, 46–47, 49, 56, 67
  in managed care, 31–32
Risk pools, 47, 48–49, 54, 56, 69
  as capitation incentives, 77–78, 90, 157
  and shared savings, 98
Riverside Hospital (OH), 142
Riverside Medical Center, 97
Riverview Hospital (IN), 109
Rocky Mountain HealthCare, 187
Roper Hospital (SC), 220
Rural areas, 16–17, 151, 213, 223
  capitation model in, 56–57, 72
  in statewide networks, 142, 151, 152
Rush-Presbyterian-St. Luke's Medical Center (IL), 35

Sachs Group (IL), 104, 151
Sacred Heart Hospital (OR), 162
Sac-Sierra Group practice (CA), 110, 111
Saint Agnes Hospital (MD), 9
Saint Bernard Hospital (IL), 78
Saint Elizabeth Hospital (NJ), 92
Saint Francis Hospital of Evanston (IL), 78
Saint James Hospital (IL), 78

Index

Saint Joseph Healthcare System (NM), 111
  and satellite clinics, 112
  strategic alliance, 217–18
  triad-model partnership, 184
Saint Joseph's Hospital and Medical Center (AZ), 9–10, 183
Saint Luke's Hospital (MO), 10
Saint Luke's Hospital (WI), 186
Saint Lukes Medical Center (OH), 142
Saint Mary of Nazareth HealthCare Network (IL), 78
Saint Mary's Hospital (NY), 112
Saint Mary's Hospital (WI), 186
Saint Paul–Ramsey Hospital (MN), 221
Saint Vincent HealthSource (AR), 191
Saint Vincent Hospital and Health Care System (IN), 8
Samaritan Health System (AZ), 92, 215, 219–20
Sanus Health Systems (NY), 29
Schlageter, Rita, 26
Schultz, Donald, 116
Scott, Richard, 141, 212
Scott and White Clinic, 52–53
Scripps (CA), 12
Scroggins, David, 53
SecureCare (IA), 215
Secure Horizons, PacifiCare, 56
Sentara Health Systems (VA), 91
Set-asides, 47

Sharp HealthCare (CA), 212, 215
  integrated delivery systems, 139–40
Sheldon, Alan, 164
Shortell, Stephen M., 202
Simone, Bridget, 186
Sisters of Mercy Health (MI), 93, 145
Sisters of Providence Health System, 34, 110, 201, 217
"Six-year insurance cycle," 27
Sklar, Joel, 152
SMG Marketing Group, 210
Sokolov, Jacques J., 143–44
Southeastern group, 187
Southern California Edison, 158
Specialists, 10–11, 45, 82–83, 90, 116
  alienation of, 133
  capitation for, 44, 48–49, 64–65
  declining income for, 96, 210
  in group practices, 128
  in HMO agreements, 125, 162
  in referral panel, 54
Specialists, referrals to, 64–65, 77, 97, 102, 130
  for Medicaid managed care, 25
  protocols for, 161
  rewards for reducing, 42, 54
  subcapitated, 47
  reimbursement for, 45, 76
  in statewide networks, 144
  surplus of, 102, 110
  See also Subspecialists
Specialty services, 146, 156, *180*, 181
  as carveouts, 69–70
  clinical prestige in, 157

Index

Spectra Health System (AZ), 88
Spivey, Bruce, M.D., 140
Spot-market contracting, 67–68, 74
Sprenger, Gordon M., 203
Springer, Gordon, 36
SSM Health Care System (MO), 142
Staff, managed care, 73
Staff-model:
  HMOs, 144–45, 182, 213–14, 217
  medical groups, 154, 156
Stanford University (CA), 161, 225
Stop-loss protection, 48, 54, 84
St. Vincent Infirmary Medical Center (AR), 191
Subcapitation, 43, 47, 49, 68–69, 74
  for centers of excellence, 161
  hospital, 68–69
Subspecialists, 75
Substance abuse services, 47, 69
Suburban Hospital Group (IN), 109
Sullivan, Michael, 189
Summit, 141, 213
Summit Care (CA), 156
Supermajority provisions, 204, 205
Suppliers, 2, 13, 134, 192
  and decreased demand, 38, 175
  and network knowledge, 18, 99
  and standardization, 59
Surgical procedures, 46, 77, *102*

Sutter Health System (CA), 12, 110, 111, 140, 183, 212
Swedish Health Services (OR), 34
Symmes Hospital (MA), 147

Teams, multifunctional, 205
Technology, 17, 90, 91, 104
  high-overhead service, 15, 167, 180
  See also Information systems
Telephone triage, 76, 107
Tenet Healthcare (TX), 146, 213, 220
  on stock exchange, 200
TennCare (TN), 148–49
Texas Oncology, 144
Third party:
  administrators, 145
  contract negotiations, 129
  intermediaries, 85
  payers, 154
  purchasers, 132
  review, 73, 79, 89, 121, 124, 162, 181
Thomas, Bill, 84
Total Quality Management/Continuous Quality Improvement, 94, 146
Travelers (CT), 32, *33*, 190
Treatment, patient:
  denial of, 7, 24, 57, 89, 121
  See also Protocols, medical
Treatment authorizations, 4, 124
Trenowski, Bernard, 187
Trust, mutual, 50, 165–66
Tucson Medical Center (AZ), 36
Tufts Associated Health Plans, 126
Tulane University (LA), 142

Ummel, Stephen L., 158, 215

Index

Underwriting, *180*
Unihealth (CA), 12, 103
United Healthcare (MN), 5, *33*, 190
  cash reserves of, 32
  expansion of, 62
  mergers, 222
  and micromanagement, 29
  and multi-year contracts, 217
  on stock exchange, 27
  and physician clinics, 35
United HealthCare Network (IL), 78
United Medical Group, 126
UnitedPhysicians (WA), 34
U.S. Healthcare (PA), 27, 32, *33*, 88
  expansion of, 62
  and micromanagement, 29
  and provider resistance, 37
UNIVA (KY), 140
University Hospitals Health System (OH), 185
University Medical Center (OH), 198
University of Chicago Medical Center, 189
University of Kansas Medical Center, 219
University of Massachusetts, 190
University of Michigan, 97
University of Minnesota Hospital, 97–98, 221, 222
University of Missouri, 97
University of Pennsylvania, 91
University of South Carolina Medical Center, 6–7
Unland, James J., 218
Utilization management, *28*, 31, 32, 37, *46*, 73, 77–78
  by provider, 49, 51, 56, 59, 84, 86, 89, *180*
  costs of, 15, 181
  in-house, 140
  programs for, 66, 89
Utilization rates, 215, 224
  decrease in, 15, 28, 44–46
Utilization review, 37, 128, 129

Valentine, Steve, 103
van Pelt, Greg, 110
Venable, Steve, 93
Vencor (KY), 147
Vertical integration, 127, 205
Virginia Mason Clinic (OR), 91, 125, 211
  in strategic alliance, 124, 201
Vision, shared, 18, 124, 205–06, 217
Vision care, 69
Voluntary Hospitals of America (TN), 99, 182–83, 207

Wasserstein, Paul, 143, 143
Wellness plan, 218–19
Wellpoint (CA), *33*
  capital reserves of, 15, 32
Westerhoff, Carl, 66
Wetzell, Steve, 86
Winter Park Memorial Hospital (FL), 213
Withholds. *See* Set-asides
Women's Hospital (MS), 189
Wyeth Insurance Company (GA), 65–66

Yedidia, Peter, 58
Yorty, John, 164

Zimmer, Daniel, 88
Zytkoskee, Adrian, 138

251

About the Author

RUSSELL C. COILE, JR., M.B.A., is a futurist specializing in the health industry. He is the president of the Health Forecasting Group, based in Dallas, Texas, and is the national strategy advisor for Chi Systems, based in Ann Arbor, Michigan. As an independent consultant, he provides market forecasts and strategic advice to a wide range of U.S. hospitals, medical groups, managed care organizations, and suppliers.

He is the author of four books in the past ten years on the future of the health field. His monthly newsletter, *Russ Coile's Health Trends,* is now in its eighth year, and his prediction rate on last year's "Top Ten Trends" was 90% accurate.

In the past year he has participated in over 100 seminars for groups including the American Hospital Association, American College of Physician Executives, the Governance Institute, and Rand Healthcare Roundtable. He is a member of the editorial advisory boards of *Managed Care Outlook, Healthcare Systems Strategy Report, Nurse Week,* and the *Medical Network Strategy Report.*

Mr. Coile holds a B.A. degree from Johns Hopkins University and an M.B.A. in Health Services Administration from George Washington University.